AYURVEDA
&LIFE IMPRESSIONS
BODYWORK

Critical Reviews of
Ayurveda & Life Impressions Bodywork

"Van is one of the few gifted teachers and healers who has distilled the best from all the bodywork systems into a process that brings about a true change in the individual."

Elizer Ben-Joseph
Herbs for Health

"This wonderful book reflects the man and his lifetime body of working wisdom in the healing arts. Like the man, it is insightful, profound, transformative, life changing, wise. Its greatest gift is its clear simplicity."

David Ford
Five Element Acupuncturist

"A must for all those who recognize Karma's role in health and healing."

Lucinda J. Dykes, M.D.

"Not only is this book a must for any bodyworker or somatic therapist, it demonstrates a way for each of us to live in our bodies with greater understanding, health, intimacy and grace."

Dr. Robert D. Waterman
President Emeritus of Southwestern College

"Van has made a journey across both time and experience to reach his profound understanding of the body, and the fruit of that journey is offered in the pages of this book."

Terry Venerable
Bodywork Therapist

"For more than a decade Donald VanHowten has been my primary source for bodywork. I credit much of my health and sense of well-being to the mastery of his subtle ministrations."

Phyllis Montgomery
Client

AYURVEDA &LIFE IMPRESSIONS BODYWORK

SEEKING OUR HEALING MEMORIES

Donald VanHowten

LOTUS

Editor and Photographs – Parvati Markus
Photographs – David Hoptman
Cover Design – Paul Bond, Art & Soul Design
Cover Illustration – Lewisa Goggin
Design and Page Layout – Carola Höchst-Teague

First Edition 1997

Printed in the United States of America

Library of Congress Cataloging-in-Publication-Data
Donald VanHowten 1948
Ayurveda and Life Impressions Bodywork:
   Seeking our Healing Memories by Donald VanHowten
   includes bibliographical references
ISBN: 0-914955-24-1   96-79622
                                                        CIP

Published by
Lotus Press, P.O. Box 325, Twin Lakes, Wisconsins 53181

Dedication

I humbly dedicate this work to my spiritual teacher,

Paramahansa Yogananda,

whose love and inspiration continually challenge

me to look carefully at my own impressions of life.

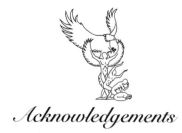

Acknowledgements

First and foremost, I give thanks to God and my spiritual teacher, Paramahansa Yogananda, for the inspiration, energy and love to complete this task.

Thanks to my family, my wife Corina, my son Talon, and my parents for their support and inspiration.

Thanks to my many wonderful teachers: Dr. Jack Painter, for his example and encouragement to treat the person, not just the body; Dr. Jerome Rosner, who reminded me I knew more than I thought I did; Eliezer Ben-Joseph for the training in touch and the elements in the body; Dr. Vasant Lad for his priceless teachings in Ayurvedic medicine and his continuing friendship; Ron Kurtz for showing me that emotional transition can be a safe rewarding adventure; Dr. John Upledger, for having the courage to share his work with people outside his profession; and Dr. Rolf, Dr. Stone, Dr. Feldenkrais and the many others who have influenced my work, although I never met them while they were alive.

I would like to offer my thanks to Hari Dev, who first inspired me regarding Ayurvedic Medicine, in the billiard room on San Francisco Street in Santa Fe...and continues to inspire, with his occasional calls from Boston when I least expect them.

I would like to thank the many students, clients, and friends who were in some way my best teachers and encouraged me in this work.

Thanks to Lenny Blank at Lotus Press for his patience and belief in this book.

Lastly, I wish to thank my Editor and friend Parvati Markus, whose contribution to this book was invaluable.

Ayurveda & Life Impressions Bodywork

TABLE OF CONTENTS

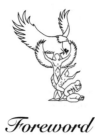

Foreword

It gives me great joy to write the foreword to this excellent book, *Ayurveda and Life Impressions Bodywork*, written by my humble, loving friend, Donald VanHowten. In this book he gives simple techniques of seeking our healing memories through Ayurvedic principles along with physical mechanics. One can clearly see in his writing the graceful blessings of Paramahansa Shri Yogandanandaji Maharaj. I have known Van since 1979, as a colleague at the Santa Fe College of Natural Medicine and in 1981 at the Institute of Traditional Medicine in Santa Fe, New Mexico.

In this book, Van brings to the reader the ancient Vedic system of healing, called Ayurveda. Ayurveda, "The Science of Life," has served humanity continuously since time immemorial and is practiced today throughout the world, especially in India, Tibet and South Asia. Ayurveda is not just a system of standardized therapeutics based upon statistical and chemical analysis of herbal medicaments, but is based upon each individual's unique constitution and imbalances. Ayurveda addresses every individual separately through proper diet, lifestyle, cleansing program of pancha karma and unique rejuvenational therapy based upon the individual's unique body type, psychological makeup, and imbalances. This practical science is based upon fundamental principles rooted in the oldest Hindu scriptures of the Atharva Veda. Ayurveda is an encyclopedia of ancient medical wisdom, natural laws and hidden secrets of long life.

Donald VanHowten has incorporated and integrated the basic principles of Ayurveda into this excellent work on connective tissue polarity. In this work he has used the word "membrane" which is similar to the Ayurvedic term kala. Kala is the boundary, the border between the two dhatus (tissues). It is the seat of datu agni (biological heat), the root of the srotas (channels) and it governs the nutrition of all bodily tissues. Kala is also the seat of ojas (immune function), tejas (the fire component), and prana (the flow of cellular intelligence). Individual mind flows through these kalas and they are the seat of subconscious memory. All of our subconscious pain, unresolved emotions, and psychological images are recorded and stored in these kalas.

In this book, Van shows that all our impressions are imprinted upon these membranes, which are responsible for many of our present sufferings and illnesses. He then demonstrates simple ways of balancing the various energy patterns that move through these membranes. He teaches us the art of reading the body's language, and methods of dealing with and healing these subconscious unresolved emotions in order to re-establish the balance between the body, mind, and consciousness.

Van is a most compassionate healer and wonderful teacher. You will love his work, expressed through this book, *Ayurveda and Life Impressions Bodywork*. Let this book be a guide to your own self-healing.

Love and Light,

Dr. Vasant Lad M.A.Sc.
Ayurvedic Physician
May, 1996

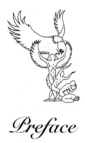

Preface

One very early morning a number of years ago, while traveling with Anandi Ma, a holy woman, and her disciples, I sat in the inner sanctum of a candle-lit temple in the Himalayan mountains. Seven Brahmin priests chanted in Sanskrit, incense perfumed the air, and smoke wafted around the giant stone lingam* in the middle of the chamber. It was a cave in which the rocks were imbued with the vibrations from many such ceremonies over thousands of years. As the prayers continued, I began to see Sanskrit symbols in my inner vision. Years before, Dr. Lad had introduced his Ayurvedic students to this ancient spiritually-based language, but I had no idea what the symbols meant.

I went deeper in my meditation. An image began to appear in my inner vision of a baby elephant, playfully swinging his trunk side-to-side. The clearer it became, the better I felt, but I had no idea what this meant or who this was. Finally I recognized that this was Ganesha, the great elephant god about whom Dr. Lad had often spoken in class. During that time we even offered a prayer to this Hindu deity each morning, but during those times I usually thought about Jesus, as I had for my whole life. I thought Hindu mythology was not for a person like myself; maybe it was a great story but... All this went through my mind in a split second and then the image was gone, leaving me with a lingering uplifting vibration along with thoughts of my own unworthiness to receive this type of vision. But despite my inner mental dialogue of "Not me,"

"Ah, shucks," and "This can't be real," I could not deny my feeling that this had been a profound blessing. Afterwards I recalled what Dr. Lad had told me about Ganesha. He is the remover of obstacles, the representation of wisdom and many other things, and this idea of "the remover of obstacles" kept returning to my mind.

Here I am, years later, still deeply entrenched in my love for my spiritual teacher Yogananda and the line of holy beings in that lineage, including the lord Jesus, Krishna, Babaji, Sri Yukteshwar, and Lahiri Mahasaya. One other follows me around my home and literally resides in me through a tattoo on my foot the elephant god Ganesha. Why the extra blessing of this wondrous being, when I am so well-guided by my lineage of teachers? One day I realized that I had been working in the field of body work and personal development for 25 years, helping people remove their obstacles. What better symbol than Ganesha, worshiped for thousands of years for just that type of work!

In India, before beginning any worthwhile task, one asks for the blessings of Ganesha. With all the love in my heart, I ask for his blessings along with those of my teacher Yogananda and the saints and sages. It is my desire that the information in this work inspire trust in your inner wisdom, awaken and spiritualize your body, mind and soul, and help to remove your obstacles.

---

* spiritual phallic symbol of the god Shiva

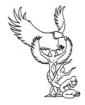

Introduction

WHAT IS LIFE IMPRESSIONS WORK?

Do you ever catch yourself holding your shoulders up for no apparent reason? When you drop your shoulders again, the forthcoming sense of relief could be called resting in neutral a state of physical, mental, and/or emotional ease. In an automobile, neutral is a place to idle, to let the engine rest before the next shift into gear, a space that allows the linkage to ease its strain. Our body tissues need that same neutral resting place. If we are frequently "uptight" and lift our shoulders in an habitual response pattern, we send a message to our shoulders to "hold tight." Our shoulders lay claim to the energy in our body and we may have trouble when the time comes to rest or sleep.

We all have holding patterns that are so habitual, ones we have repeated so often throughout our lives that they literally leave an historic imprint on the membranes of the body, which are the connective tissues that hold everything else inside us in place. These membranes store our repetitive actions and experiences, along with our solidified emotions and ideas, as life impressions.

The purpose of Life Impressions work is to help us become who we really are. Although this sounds like a cosmic statement, it is actually a practical application. Through proper understanding of who we are and how we can change mentally, emotionally, elementally, and physically we can learn to release those life impressions that bind us. We can increase our flexibility in both behavior and body function. Therapists can use the gentle, non-invasive, membrane-release techniques given in this book to aid in developing the safety and support needed for change. We can update our historic imprints, release the stored healing memories, and improve our lives.

We carry in our minds and bodies all the events of our personal histories. Some of this history is still relevant to our present-day lives, but some of it is quite outdated, which leaves us stuck both in our beliefs and our membranes. We then function and behave according to an old self-image based on who we used to be.

Let's say you severely sprained your right ankle ten years ago; subconsciously you may feel insecure about running from danger. Maybe you had a complexion problem back in high school and twenty years later still sport a beard to cover up the marks. Maybe you were embarrassed when you couldn't answer questions in class and still feel you aren't intelligent or can't speak in a group. In truth, we are no longer the same people who experienced those original events. However, not only do we carry around these barnacles imbedded in our flanks, but we tend to run our lives under their influence. By freeing that ankle so we know it can support us, by increasing personal safety to the point where we can risk shaving the beard or speaking to a group, we are able to become more of who we really are.

Life Impressions work is designed to release safely the historic imprints held in our bodies. We use the Touch of Awakening to liberate the healing memories and loosen the potential freedom compacted in the life impressions. Life Impressions work awakens the information and support, and offers safe practical skills needed to "drop our shoulders" and be at peace within.

WHO CAN USE THIS INFORMATION?

The information in this book is for anyone who is seeking to live life with true ease and suspects the answers may lie within. The massage therapist, rolfer, physical therapist, Ayurvedic therapist or any other therapist willing to explore new methods for treating old problems will also find new information here.

The ideas behind Life Impressions can aid doctors who feel there is something more than just the chemical, biological, mechanical and physiological world of medicine, doctors who may have witnessed unexplained healing in patients. It is for those who know that listening to the patient and getting the patient involved in his/her own treatment is a vital part of the healing process. This is for the physician who understands that touch, even a simple heartfelt pat on the shoulder to a trusting patient, conveys more than just pressure and summons forth more than just a sensory response.

Mental health professionals can make more meaningful, clear contact with their patients. Therapists who see that feelings are expressed by bodies as well as words, therapists who see self-image reflected in behavior and wonder about the "coincidence" of similar body-types behaving in a similar fashion all can benefit.

Life Impressions work is for anyone who understands there is a connection between our external and internal environments, and that our health is established or destroyed through our food, our feelings, and our actions. For each person who wants to be involved in his own growth and healing and/or to help friends and loved ones, this book offers specific therapeutic understanding and practical application techniques for a new way of communicating, for acknowledging that we are spiritual beings with feelings that are sometimes uncomfortable and with bodies that sometimes hurt.

BENEFITS

If we read and respond to the history that is imprinted in our tissues, we begin the process of change and liberation. In the case of therapists, we assist our patients in discovering ways to make lasting changes, not through analysis and manipulation, but by helping them to seek the healing memories within and update their self-image on all levels neurologically, emotionally, and physically.

There is an old East Indian proverb: You can feed a beggar one day and he will be hungry again the next; if you teach the beggar to grow his own food, he will be fed for a long time to come. All change is preceded by increased awareness. When the message comes from inside ourselves and has been reinforced with practical experience, we can sustain change. We cannot change our attitude without a corresponding body response; we cannot change body function or shape without the attitude changing.

Dis-ease can be viewed as a symbol, an expression or attitude of the mind and body that is not congruent with our true nature. In the over-stressed lives many of us lead, the life-force is being mishandled. If we learn to balance the forces in our life, we may no longer need to overindulge in pain relievers of many kinds. All the treatment methods in Life Impressions work are designed first to increase awareness and second to assist the reordering of the personal system under the guidance of the client's inner wisdom. With the information available in Life Impressions, we have the opportunity to become who we really are, free of the historic imprints, free from the old images of our self and our self-created bindings.

EAST MEETS WEST

Most treatment systems today are usually presented through an exclusively Western viewpoint, while Eastern methods have been designated as alternative or complementary venues. I feel that it is far more effective to take the best from each and to use the two systems together. Like my spiritual teacher, Paramahansa Yogananda, I feel that a deeper understanding takes place when East meets West. This book is my opportunity to take the wisdom from the East, specifically from the ancient science of Ayurvedic medicine, mix it with a version of the Western medical model, stir in large portions of awareness, safety, and support, add practical healing techniques, and pass the recipe along into capable hands and hearts.

To offer this kind of personalized work, we must understand human nature, looking deeper than the nuts and bolts of anatomy into the elemental level of human beings. People change from moment to moment, season to season, literally with every thought, and these changes have to be taken into account during treatment. Knowing how to contact a person in the appropriate manner requires profound insight, which can be enhanced through the study of the Eastern science of Ayurvedic medicine.

BOOK STRUCTURE

Section I "Who Are We?" offers new ways of looking at ourselves. Chapter One shows how a Life Impression is made, how the body develops physical, emotional, and mental historic imprints. Here, and throughout the book, simple exercises are provided which give the reader an experiential knowledge of the information. A basic introduction to Ayurvedic principles in Chapter Two gives enough background for us to see ourselves from a new perspective. To quote Dr. Lad, the eminent Ayurvedic doctor, we learn to read the "living book." Chapter Three explores our self-image based on our interactions with the inner and outer environments. Chapter Four is a thorough explanation of the function of the membranes.

The information in these early chapters allows us to see ourselves and others in a new and different light, and develops our respect for the diversity of physical, emotional, and mental types.

Section II "How We Change" contains useful information on recognizing the need for change and how to go about it. Chapter Five introduces the technique of the Touch of Awakening. The essential relationship of all component parts is explored in Chapter Six. Chapter Seven discusses intervention through the Touch of Awakening.

General treatments are offered in Section III "Treatments and Resources" which can be used by anyone willing to listen sensitively to the needs of another person. Vital Air, Component, and Elemental Treatments (Chapters Eight-Ten), although general and non-invasive, are very effective by themselves or together with other work. More complex treatment techniques are indicated for therapists. All are safe. A list of resources for further information and continuing education follows.

SECTION I

Who Are We?

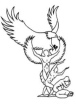

Chapter One

The Making of a Life Impression

Be careful what you choose to do consciously,
for unless your will is very strong,
that is what you may have to do repeatedly.

-Paramahansa Yogananda

It's a hot summer day and you're sitting out on the porch in your shorts in one of those wrought iron chairs made with little criss-cross patterns so water can drain through the holes. After a while, you get up and wander back into the house. Your friend, walking behind you, is laughing, "Hey, the back of your legs look like a waffle iron!" Sure enough, you're carrying an impression made by the chair and, depending on circumstances, you may feel amused, embarrassed, or annoyed. Life has been impressed in your flesh.

Sometimes the impressions made on us by life are initiated by such simple physical events, but often life impressions are first established from a mental or emotional situation and then become physical. Our parents are yelling at each other again, our heart aches, and we collapse our chests in a protective gesture around our heart. If the hurt continues or we're re-injured later on, the pattern of protection increases in intensity and density and becomes established as a life impression. The dents in our legs imprinted by the porch chair will go away quickly, but our collapsed chest may become a deeply rooted part of our physical make-up, supported by an image of ourselves that comes from a much earlier time in our life.

What would happen if you added financial worries or brought some family conflict to the chair and then sat on it all day for many months? Our thoughts and feelings are not just in our heads and hearts; whatever we are experiencing in life is contained throughout the organism. If we sat in the chair, establishing the chair imprint, and then added some inner turmoil, we would develop both physical and emotional imprints.

As a young child, Dave was playing with a dog which ran into the street and was killed by a car. Dave was devastated. His ribs closed up from sobbing, and the intensity of feeling produced a "stickum" (a technical term) which kept the ribs in their contracted state. The event was stored in the contracted ribs and life went on. As a teenager, Dave met a young lady and fell in love, then she and her family moved away. Because young men aren't supposed to cry, Dave clamped down on his feelings, which produced more stickum and further glued down his ribs. As other events accumulated, they solidified the life impression for Dave: don't let the feeling escape, keep the ribs contracted, don't get involved, don't let your love out or you'll be overwhelmed by grief and embarrassed by crying. The contracted rib pattern was charged again and again with deepening grief; his experience became etched in flesh.

Finally, Dave met his one true love. She said, "Why can't you open up to me?"

The young man insisted, "I am, I am," but deep inside his stuck-together ribs, his heart was saying, "Not with your impression of life, no way!"

In Dave's case, the stickum and the bindings that hold back the feelings are the first barriers to loosening the stuck ribs. Dave needs to discover the hidden healing memory, the action that could help heal his pain, which for him would be to cry.

He was unwilling or unable to cry after the first experience with his dog's death. Those tears are still on hold, gluing down his ribs. If he could allow himself to feel his accumulated grief, Dave would experience some healing.

Dave desperately wants to change so his true love will know his feelings, but how? How do we initiate lasting change, bring ourselves more in line with the joy of living? Consider how easily we can change our minds. A brief shift in thought and we have made a major decision: Yes, today I start my diet. But how difficult is it to follow through on that decision? It's like trekking through the forest: first you blaze the trail, then the next time you find the path and repeat the journey, making a groove. Once the path is well-established and the vegetation has grown thick around your chosen path, it becomes hard to deviate from that route. Even after the mind makes a solid choice to change, the established routes in the nervous system and the physical body must be re-patterned.

When I was working in Sweden, I asked a friend who often traveled to the far north of the country what it was like there in the winter. He told about driving to visit his relatives when the snow was many feet high along the sides of the road. After coming to a sudden stop, his car began to do several 360 degree turns. When he finally came to rest, he looked in both directions and saw nothing but a tunnel of snow. Disoriented, not knowing which way to go, he picked a direction and ended up going back to the city he had just left. The same limitations develop in our life as we become patterned by our life impressions, the tunnels become defined and we behave like a train on a set of tracks with few options. Dave may want to open up, to share his feelings, but his entrenched impressions won't let him.

11

Etched in Flesh

No matter whether they were initiated by physical, mental or emotional causes, life impressions become etched into our flesh because they become established in the membranes the thin, soft layers of connective tissue that cover or line an organ, bone, muscle or other body part. The human body is literally held together by the membranes. In fact, all aspects of the organism have a container or membrane which serves as a boundary, as a way of separating one body part from another or keeping our insides separate from the outside world around us. Membranes must separate the chambers of the heart or it will not pump properly. Divisions are needed between the muscle groups in order for the muscles to do their work. If the membranes stick to one another or become hardened, their efficiency drops and they can no longer maintain integrity between various components of the system.

Not only do the membranes create our boundaries, they also move the fluids in our bodies by functioning like hydraulic pumps. As we move, large and small membrane sheets slide against one another, often going in different directions, moving the fluids that are between the membranes. The human body is composed primarily of fluids which have many different tasks: the blood carries nourishment, the nerve fluid carries electrical stimuli and information, some fluids carry immune material, others lubricate and reduce friction. Such a large mass of liquid must be contained and kept moving if we are to avoid becoming watery blobs rolling from place to place.

The membranes also provide the bedding for our nerves. They carry information from place to place in the body because nerve fibers permeate the membranes. We communicate from toe to head through that network of nerve endings, laced together by the connective tissue membranes which hold the nerve roots in place.

In the formation of a life impression, the membranes are the clay upon which information is etched. When you sat on the porch chair, the fluids between the layers of tissue were separated into the patterned sections of flesh and were temporarily held in place by the membrane system, leaving you impressed from the outside in. The membranes support the shape we impose on ourselves, whether from the inside out or the outside in, because their main job is safety and support. Dave's emotional reaction to his little puppy's death wasn't originally a physical imprint, but it became physical because Dave protected his aching heart by clamping down his ribs.

Dave spent much of his adult life walking around scrunched over, protecting his heart. He wondered why he couldn't sustain a relationship, couldn't stay open to a loved-one. He attended workshops on the emotions and went into therapy through which he developed insight into his historic information. "No wonder I behave this way, look at what happened to me! Wow! Now I just feel great." Then someone else tried to get close to him and that old membrane memory reasserted itself. "Oh, geez. Back again," scrunched over protectively. Even with the mental insight in place, his body was still holding on to the old historic imprint.

Imagine walking down the beach looking out at the ocean. A very wonderful day has passed and the sun is going down. All of a sudden the wind picks up and shakes a palm tree, loosening a coconut which hits you on the head. You're open and receptive, everything is really beautiful, then Clunk! Your body says, "Wow. I can't afford to be that open. It's dangerous." The nerves in the membranes record the information. The membranes harden a little.

13

Time passes. You forget the incident, but your body doesn't. It's an interesting thing about bodies: they don't have a relationship to time and space; time and space are creations of the mind. As far as the body is concerned, you just got hit on the head with the coconut today. All the pain and anguish and tears encapsulated in the membranes are waiting. Twenty years later you're walking along on another beach when you see a palm tree. It's very unlikely that another coconut is going to bean you, but your body doesn't know that because the pain of the previous experience is still held in the tissues. Your body is on guard for signals that recall that incident the beach, the tree, the sea breeze are all pleasurable sensory experiences, but that old historic imprint automatically remembers the coconut and won't let you relax. Until the life impression is released from the tissues, it can continue to reappear when a situation jogs your membrane memory.

FOCUSING AWARENESS

Dave had an emotional impact, but his membranes got stuck on it; he wants his heart to be open, but his chest hurts every time he gets a lover in his life. At least part of that pain is because Dave can't get his old puppy and girlfriend experiences out of his chest. To free himself from the historic impressions, Dave needs increased awareness of the situation and physical freedom from the membrane restrictions that hold the memories in his body. To attain the physical freedom, he needs a sense of safety and support. The physical life impression needs to be addressed so he can get on with his life.

If we are to be truly happy and to function well in our lives, we need to look deeply within ourselves, conduct regular search and rescue operations, and if need be, reorganize ourselves. However, when there has been a major event, such as an injury to the body, the membranes of the traumatized area tend to thicken and build a wall of protection which isolates the area from the rest of the system. The thickening can interfere with the nerves that are woven through the tissues like the roots of a plant. The nerves are an avenue for our awareness to travel from place to place within us. The intelligence or information within the nerves responds to our need for protection and support and the tissues become stiffer and thicker, or softer and more yielding, depending on what is needed.

When the membranes of an injured area become too thick, it becomes harder for the nerves to carry clear messages throughout the system. We literally begin to "lose touch" with areas of our body when the signals are unclear, muffled by the membranes. We can no longer easily access information from the injured area because we can't feel it as well as we used to and, in some cases, we cannot even locate the area. If the injured area is well-protected, we may not even know it's missing and/or dysfunctional. We need to reclaim these lost areas to get back our functional potential. The only way to retrieve the lost function is to first increase awareness, "highlighting" the area in our attention through a technique such as Touch of Awakening (Chapter Five).

All the cells and tissues in our bodies are full of consciousness. Prana a Sanskrit word meaning the force of life at its subtlest level is pure consciousness and, as such, is present in every cell of the human body. Awakening to the need for change, even the initial notice of the need for change can begin the physical meltdown of membrane blocks, releasing clear information and the ability to act. We can stimulate the membranes to reorganize so they can provide the support and safety we need, giving us back our functionality and expanding our personal options.

For example, all the delicate articulations between the heel and toes of a foot are often lost from so many years of wearing shoes and socks. We no longer have any awareness of these articulations; they are no longer in our picture of ourselves. If we can get those articulations out of storage, we can relieve the strain on the rest of the foot structure and the joint capsules of the knee, the ankle, the hip and so on. We need to learn how to actively mobilize the missing parts so that the neurology, the kinesthetic sense of our body, can pick up on the articulations. "Wow! I didn't know my foot was supposed to move that way!"

Every one of us has a large number of possible action patterns that have never been used before and remain therefore entirely foreign...

-Moshe Feldenkrais

Think about your hands for a moment, how many tasks they do every day, year after year. The hands are often the first of our body parts to touch the world around us; therefore they encounter difficulties that the rest of us are glad to have avoided. We touch to see if something is hot; we feel around in the dark for an object. The hands are very sensitive and are acutely aware of the possibility of danger, particularly after a few mishaps. With these ideas in mind, we can already assume there are some historically-imprinted experiences in our hands.

Now consider the repetitive experiences in your hands. How many times have you turned a door knob the same way? What about all those years of writing, or typing? Your hands have done many actions many times with the exact same timing and manner. You probably worked long and hard to get those useful patterns in place, but what about all the options that are ruled out by the habitual pattern?

The following exercise is designed to help bring awareness to your hands and to rediscover your options for their use. It is helpful to have someone read this to you or record it.

Exercise:

Rediscover Your Hands

Sit comfortably at a desk, with your eyes closed and your hands resting on the desk top or your knees, palms down. Notice your right hand. Is it relaxed, stiff, or some of each in different areas?

Notice the fingers (still with your eyes closed, you gain more information this way). Are they straight or slightly bent? Can you feel the entire length of the fingers or just the part in contact with the desk? How does your palm feel? Does it rest flat on the desk or is it pressed in on one corner with the other edge slightly lifted off the desk surface?

Lift only your right index finger 1/16th of an inch and then let it down. Do this several times. (Just notice how it moves; don't try to make something happen. You are adding information to the system, not trying to fix or change anything. Change often comes from the increased awareness of what you do, but please wait for that to emerge.) Let the hand rest and notice any changes. Now lift the middle finger many times, only 1/16th of an inch. Rest and feel any change. Then move the ring finger, the little finger, and finally the thumb.

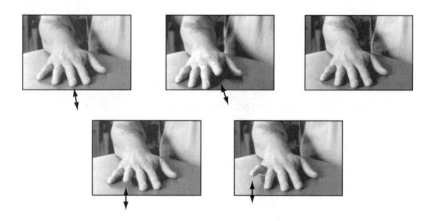

Now imagine there is a ball in your palm. Keeping your fingers at rest, slightly lift the heel of your hand as if you were going to roll across the ball toward your index finger and back, slowly and only a very short distance, several times. Rest, then roll across the imaginary ball toward the middle finger several times. Then the ring finger, the little finger, and then the thumb.

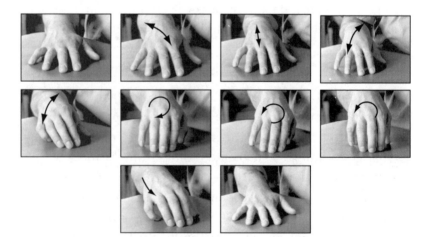

Compare your hands. Move them around gently, feel the lightness. Place them back on your desk or lap. Again, with the right hand, imagine the ball in your palm. Begin to roll around the ball outwardly, slowly and many times. Allow your right shoulder to participate in the rolling. Reverse the direction and roll a number of times. Can you feel any movement in your ribs?

You have completed one hand. Notice the changes, not just in the hand, but in the whole self. Slowly move your arms, your neck. Open your eyes and walk around, noting differences in how you feel. Compare the two sides of your body. Try the other hand.

Through using yourself in a different way, you are creating more awareness of your options and changing the pattern and consistency of the tissues of your hand. You may have reduced your historic imprinting in that simple exercise. Whatever change you did note, the growth has begun; you now have more options in your brain and body. Another interesting fact to consider is that you have started learning from your own organism. This type of learning is not bound by the hard edges of medical or scientific volumes, but is free to grow from within in all directions.

How Membranes Respond

The nerves that are embedded within the membranes respond to challenges, our perception of safety, and the beliefs we have built up within ourselves. Membranes can react very spontaneously or with a very patterned response when the nerves call the membranes into action.

Imagine lying in your crib as an infant. I like to go back to this level because at that stage in our lives we moved and responded very spontaneously, with very few preconceived patterns and without the musculature to do something through our own effort. One side of your crib is up against a barren wall; on the other side a mobile is spinning and across the room is the door where Mom and Dad and Brother enter from time to time. Obviously, your curiosity and spontaneity are more often focused to the side that is more interesting. If you keep directing your attention toward the interesting side, your eyes begin to organize, or pattern themselves better in that direction. Soon the neck and head organize in that direction. It's not a calculated thing. There is no analytical involvement. There is no agenda. It happens because your preference is organically developing around spontaneity and curiosity and your orientation in that direction becomes very efficient. For better or worse, an early life impression has been created.

Mom has become an interesting figure in your life. Maybe you have even organized your self-image around, "Oh, she does this with me and makes me do this and that." In short, you think you are now someone in relation to someone else, and have a personal relationship to the environment around you which includes this special person, "Mom." She walks away and comes back, walks away and comes back, doing her daily tasks. You assume that her world has to do with you alone. You follow her actions with your eyes to a point where not only your neck has oriented to her actions, but also your chest is now starting to organize to follow her.

One day Mom walks away and you watch her to the end of your developing functional limit. All of a sudden, clunk, you're on your stomach. What a concept! You didn't calculate that body response; you discovered the possibility. You followed your curiosity about Mom until your brain and nervous system organized your body to function in a new manner. It's a positive historic imprint, but it works best in one direction. At this point you are "softly organized." You can still change. You have, as Moshe Feldenkrais would say, "reversible movement." This reversibility, or ability to "undo" ourselves, is what we seek when we free ourselves from unwanted life impressions or historic imprints. We want to get back to being a flexible non-patterned person who has choices.

One day your parents slide the crib over to the other side of the room to clean, and they leave it there for a day or two. Now Mom's coming and going from another direction. Oh, this is not working too well, because you organized the other way and really got behind it. The pattern had "set up" in the softer elements, like gelatin in a mold, but because you are still somewhat flexible, you soon learn to follow Mom's movements from this new direction as well.

As in this crib analogy, we may find a propensity later in life to turn more easily to one side than to the other. Over time we pattern our whole organism in our unique way; maybe it doesn't work at optimum efficiency, but we get the job done. As membranes mold to a task, they often restrict our other options. The longer we stay in one physical position, the more attention we put into an action or inhibition and the more often it is repeated, the more bound we become within our self-made tissue support system. The more we see ourselves in only one way, the less available we are both functionally and in attitude to do or be something else. There is great worth in being able to view one's self from different perspectives and having the functional capability to do different things in life.

As we look at the idea of how to bring about change, we must appreciate that which has been created and learn to work with the system, not against it. We must appreciate the way our bodies have organized themselves, applaud the ingenuity of the membranes, nerves, bones, and muscles as they went about creating safety and support. If we evaluate a particular pattern as "wrong" and think it should be altered, we may create disharmony. We must look at appropriate interventions. By understanding the human organism from different perspectives, such as looking at it from the viewpoint of the ancient science of Ayurvedic medicine, we can receive and treat clients with more respect and wisdom. Later chapters in this book offer many methods of treatment which respect the wisdom expressed by the recipients body.

When we understand some of the principles of Ayurvedic medicine, we can better understand when and with whom to use a certain type of touch. To better understand the nature of the organism and our personal relationship to it, the next chapter takes us through the perspective of the science of Ayurvedic medicine. We must understand the needs of each person from various points of view inside and outside, Eastern and Western to provide a multi-dimensional update of our life impressions and allow us to enjoy a fuller, happier life.

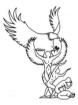

Chapter Two

The Mother of All Healing

In Sanskrit, Ayurveda means the study of life. According to ancient Hindu texts, all healing systems stem from Ayurvedic medicine. I had been practicing manual therapy and various forms of bodywork and personal development for at least thirteen years before I began to study Ayurvedic medicine with the eminent Dr. Lad in Santa Fe. It didn't seem new to me because my studies in Polarity Therapy clearly had roots in this ancient science. I soon understood that everything I had ever studied which stood the test of time also had strong ties to Ayurveda. Now, more than a dozen years later, I am still impressed by the profound wisdom of this ancient science.

Ayurvedic theory and practice have been gleaned from centuries of introspection, meditation and the experience of some of India's great sages, healers and teachers. It is not within the scope of this book to cover the vast and complex science of Ayurvedic medicine in great detail. There are profound works available on the subject (see Bibliography). Here I am presenting only a brief summary of some of the basic principles of Ayurveda which are most relevant to working with our life impressions.

If we think of ourselves primarily as a physical body, or just as an intellect to the exclusion of our emotional and physical aspects, we limit our ability to understand and respond to the changing demands of life. If, however, we can see ourselves from many different perspectives, we can learn more about who we are and respond more readily to change when it arises.

Awareness includes our perceptions of ourselves on all levels, our relationship to life. We are usually not conscious of being unaware of a complicated thought, but it is nonetheless there. Let's say you have an allergic reaction to bananas, but you don't know that. In fact, each time you get these particular symptoms, you think you have the flu and take some drug or herb, rest, maybe pray, and eventually the symptoms go away. One day you read an article about allergies and recognize the description of the symptoms. A food allergy test proves that bananas produce a strong adverse reaction in your body. Through increased awareness you have healed yourself of the "flu." What this chapter will add to your database of self-knowledge is an awareness of how the five basic elements, as described in Ayurvedic medicine, compose our bodies and affect us.

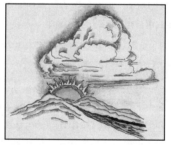

THE ELEMENTS

Although we will look at the elements from an Eastern perspective, Western science also breaks down all matter to its elemental components. What is added by Ayurveda is the way in which these elements comprise the building blocks of our constitutions and how we can use this knowledge to restore balance to our systems.

All organic and inorganic substances are composed of combinations of the basic five elements:

Space (ether) the Final Frontier. Space is the all-pervading "home" for all objects in the universe, the field from which everything is manifested and into which everything returns. When we refer to someone as being "spaced out," in reality this may be so.

In a sense, space could be considered the idea plane, the blueprint, where things are built in the mind. Lying in bed one morning, your mind drifts into thinking you are sick and overworked and need a rest. When the alarm clock goes off, you find you are stiff and achy and your throat hurts... hmm, where did that come from? The blueprint was made in the mind and you filled it in on the physical plane.

Air is the gaseous state of matter, existence without form. Air is vital for all living creatures; it is essential for establishing location in the body, such as the area between the cells in the lungs or between body parts. For structures to differentiate in function, space and air must be available or movement is impossible. For example, if the lungs become congested and fill with fluid, if the alveoli and the little lung sacs for breathing become cramped and watered down with mucus, the space and air elements have been encroached upon by water and movement in the lungs is hindered. Another example would be a swamp, which, unlike a well-drained pond, lacks the movement that the element of air produces.

Fire is the power of transformation that can convert a substance from solid to liquid to gas and vice versa; form without substance. Have you ever moved your finger through a candle flame? If so, you have direct experience of seeing the form of fire while knowing there is no substance; you moved right through the flame. The activity of fire governs digestion, absorption, and assimilation in the living organism as well as the flowering, ripening and decaying of plants. Fire is necessary to melt down congestion. If you are dieting but not losing weight, you are probably missing the fire of activity exercise produces heat that in turn burns the calories, and the tissues can then begin to melt away.

Water is the liquid state of matter whose characteristic attribute is flux; substance without stability. Water is the life-sustaining liquid, the cooling element which maintains electrolyte balance, nourishes plants and animals, and sustains the environment. Water gives grace and flow to our movements. After having a fever, we often feel stiff because the fire of the fever has burned off the water in our system and the joint capsules have dried a bit. If we soak in a warm bath and drink some nourishing liquid, we will feel more flexible.

Earth is the solid state of matter, whose characteristic attribute is stability, fixity or rigidity; stable substance. Earth is the solid, dense element which provides the firm ground for global life. Earth gives form to the body. The heavier tissues of the body, such as the connective tissues and bones, contain more earth element and thus provide the needed stability in our body for dealing with the strains and effort of life.

All five elements flow throughout the entire body, but, according to Ayurvedic medicine, there are certain areas where one or more of the particular elements dominate. The mind, for example, is composed primarily of the elements of air and ether, with the fire of intelligence and some watery memory. Mental components are very light, subtle and changeable. The body, on the other hand, is much denser, composed primarily of water and earth for strength and sustainability, some fire for warmth and processing, and some air and ether for movement.

We want to be able to change our congested, stiff, impaired

bodies into vital healthy structures. To effectively bring about something new in ourselves, we must change our idea (ether), move (air) that into the body, melt (fire) the habitual pattern in the tissues, and restore the form (water and earth). Until we can implement change in the heavier elements of the body, the mind, which shifts easily through ether and air, can't manifest the changes it wants to make. We can easily visualize the change, but to complete it we must include the body.

According to Ayurveda, there is awareness in all our tissues, which is called prana, the life-force. Since prana is present throughout the whole system, each event in our lives affects our whole body and mind. Let's look again at the waffle net imprinted on the back of our thighs by the chair. We can see that the information in the layers of flesh has been compacted by the pressure of sitting in the chair, leaving stagnation much like that in the swamp, which has no air flow and therefore little movement or vitality.

This congestion, or overcrowding of the local tissues, can be relieved by adding air and ether through movement. As you get up from the chair, the action of rising produces movement which increases space available in the tissues; the air element can enter the region and reduce the chair imprint. The stagnation could also be broken up by heat: the blood contains heat, a fire element, which warms the "squished" tissue (a technical term) by melting down the congestion caused by the chair impression. The waffle-look fades from your legs. In short, the prana is now flowing and the tissues return to normal.

Let's add another factor to the chair drama. You're young and impressionable, and out on your first double date. As you get up from the chair, wearing shorts and waffled thighs, you hear giggling and know your date is laughing at you. If you've been trying to impress your date, you're likely to react with feelings such as embarrassment, anger, or shame. Now we've added insult to the mechanical impression: an emotional charge that produces a chemical reaction, a small amount of emotional "stickum" (another technical term for collagen with emotional juice in it) is expressed into the tissue, particularly in the area of tissue disturbance, and changes the bio-mechanical action to some degree. If you become angry, the heat increases and it is likely that the tissues in the area will become red and the impression will last longer. If you're sad about what happened, the water in the body increases and the extra fluid makes the impression last longer. In other words, the elements respond to your reaction.

Now you have a complex impression; not only do you have to normalize from the chair imprint, but you have to move out the feeling as well. How well we clear the imprint depends upon our awareness of the whole process, including our feelings, and then finding a balance to the elemental order so the tissues can return to normal. If any component is not addressed, a Life Impression will remain which will bind some of our energy and awareness in that place and event.

THE THREE DOSHAS: THE CONSTITUTIONAL TYPES

Groups of elements form our feelings, body, actions, and beliefs into a pattern, called our constitution. There are three types of constitutions in the Ayurvedic system, based on the Three Doshas (principles), the various combinations of the five elements vata (air and space), pitta (fire and water) and kapha (water and earth).

At the time of conception, each person's constitution (prakruti) is created by the way in which the three doshas combine through the union of the parents. Other factors besides genetics influence the creation of constitution, such as the diet, lifestyle and emotions of the parents, and the external environment where we are conceived and under what conditions, including the weather and even the time of day. I am not referring to astrology, although the heavenly bodies do have an effect; I am referring to the elements of our own earthly environment, the environmental factors at the moment we arrive.

Let's say your parents-to-be live over a fire station and you are born as the station is mobilizing to go fight a fire. The dramatic bells and sirens elicit a definite elemental response, perhaps producing the emotions of fear and anxiety (vata), or the emotions of excitement or anger (pitta). Building upon that first day's emotional response, you may increase or decrease certain internal elements to cope with your perception of the environment.

Because of the great excitation and activity (both traits of air and ether) happening around you in those early moments, your inner elements of air and ether are likely to be increased, aggravating the nervous system. That in turn may cause you to be on edge, excitable, and highly active, traits which compose the general pattern of your life. Who knows? Maybe you chose this birthplace for those very reasons. But the fact remains that you must learn to function in life based on your beginnings. It may be that you develop a desire for more food to strengthen and solidify the system and balance the high-strung inner pattern. Perhaps you add more water to absorb some of the impact. There are any number of options. The point of understanding constitution is to learn what your tendencies are and to learn the options for balancing yourself.

Maybe you were born at home under the most pleasant and safest of circumstances. Grandma, who is a very excitable person, has been waiting anxiously to see the new arrival. One day she bursts upon the scene and, with overflowing emotion, scoops you out of your crib. This is the first time anything this powerful has happened since you were born. You draw on the elements within you to deal with this new input, organizing them into a response in the nerves and tissues. You may draw on the heavy elements, water and earth, to stiffen yourself against the experience. Generally, you will choose the most abundant elements, further enhancing your constitution and adding another historic imprint to your impressions of life on planet Earth.

Once the constitution is formed, we view life through it and must learn to create balance from there. When all three doshas are equal in quality and quantity, they produce good health and excellent digestion, and life may seem to have fewer bumps. Some people just seem to sail along, getting good grades in school without working hard, eating anything and never gaining weight, and so on. They are few and far between. My teacher Yogananda said that these people developed their qualities through the work of many earlier lives. Most of us usually have to work to stay in balance.

Basic constitution does not change during our lifetime. However, we also have a constitution of the moment, called vikruti, which reflects our present state of health. The vikruti is usually different from the prakruti, the constitution with which we are born. It is this difference that provides the Ayurvedic physician with enough information to formulate a program for restoring health.

The imbalance in our constitution is not a defect; it represents something of value, something we can work with and learn from. The majority of people, who have one or two doshas prominent, can achieve optimum health through proper diet and lifestyle, adding or reducing elemental qualities as needed. If we learn to understand our constitutions both that of inheritance and that of the moment we can deal with present symptoms and long term re-balancing. By understanding what increases and decreases the elements, and with good hands-on work, we can find relative balance within any constitution.

In essence, if we understand the dominant elements of our constitution and their attributes, we can understand how to achieve balance in our lives by avoiding what we don't need and increasing that which we are lacking. As we learn more about constitutions and what makes the elements increase and decrease, we learn how to create a favorable environment for ourselves. This is practical information. Understanding the principles and attributes of the three types of constitution will help keep us in balance, help us understand others when they are out of balance, and offer new ways to look at old problems.

In general I am not inclined to box people into categories, so take the following information as reference material, not as a label. At best this is something about you, not the real you. Don't get symptomatic from the following information. I remember sitting in classes in acupuncture and Ayurveda as we discussed one malady after another; I was sure I suffered from each disease, and on occasion temporarily developed symptoms. Discussing symptoms can be very disconcerting. Affirm your well-being as often as possible.

THE VATA (AIR) CONSTITUTION

The dosha of vata is composed of the elements of air and space/ether. Vata is mainly concerned with the nervous system and the control of all body movement. It is the principle of movement made manifest in the body. One of the best ways to understand and balance any dosha is to understand its common characteristics, qualities, or attributes. The following chart of the vata attributes shows what needs to be increased and decreased in the dosha. For example, to balance the dryness of vata one would add moist, unctuous, warm qualities.

In general, a person with a vata constitution is very mobile, quick, light in weight, dry, cold, with skin rough to the touch. Crooked structures are common due to random movements of the air and ether energies within the spine and nervous system. A balanced vata constitutional type is very light and active. The person with dominant vata characteristics is light-hearted, has a quick mind, but forgets easily, whereas an unbalanced vata type may seem weak, insecure, untrustworthy, and a bit agitating to be around. A person with too much vata will tend to have a hyperactive mind, which can produce fear and anxiety; the balanced vata person is exuberant and joyful due to the light qualities of their predominant elements.

Consider for a moment the vata attribute of mobility. To understand how an attribute can affect the constitution, examine what can happen when mobility is increased in the vata person. First of all, the vata person is mobile by nature. Increased mobility creates a specific effect inside the body: kinetic energy vitality produced as a result of motion, like rubbing your hands together and producing heat. The more a person moves about, even subtly, the more kinetic energy is produced in the body until it becomes almost self-generating.

In the vata person, inner movement in the form of mental activity, as well as general random body movement, generates more kinetic energy. At some point this energy has to leave the system or it can adversely affect the nerves and tissues. This cycle of building and dissipating energy is a general pattern. If we get stuck in building energy and don't "get it out," we become prone to nervous twitches, anxiety, even joint problems due to the energy accumulating about the joints. If the energy becomes trapped, it literally requires more energy to hold it in place, frequently resulting in depletion and a deranged vata condition.

Imagine you are watching an action movie in which the characters are going through great turmoil. Although you are sitting passively, your nervous system is reacting to the movement on the screen. Your elements respond (air and ether get off on this type of vicarious activity), excited by the mental activity and visual stimuli, and they produce energy in the system and nerve excitation; the heart rate may rise. You remain seated for two hours and build a charge. Whether or not you have a vata constitution, you have a charge inside that needs to be dissipated or utilized. If you are vata, you may have a more urgent need to do something, and possibly feel drained at the same time.

A vata type, sitting on the webbed chair, will only sustain a slight imprint because they have less of the water element. On the other hand, their excitable nature may produce a lot of energy and anxiety may arise. The factor most likely to hold the impression is the very active mind: long after the body impression has faded, the vata person may still be thinking about it.

Vata Attributes

Attributes	Manifestations in the Body
Dry	dry skin, hair, lips, tongue; dry colon, tending toward constipation; hoarse voice
Light	light muscles, bones, thin body frame, light scanty sleep; underweight
Cold	cold hands, feet, poor circulation; hates cold and loves hot; stiffness of muscles
Rough	rough, cracked skin, nails, hair, teeth, hands and feet; cracking joints
Subtle	subtle fear, anxiety, insecurity; fine goose-pimples; minute muscle twitching, fine tremors; delicate body
Mobile	fast walking, talking, doing many things at a time; restless eyes, eyebrows, hands, feet; unstable joints; many dreams; loves traveling but does not stay at one place; mood swings and shaky faith
Clear	clairvoyant; understands and forgets immediately; clear, empty mind, experiences void and loneliness

Vata body type: often slim (due to increased nervous activity and mobile qualities), although the abdomen slightly protrudes even in slim individuals because the abdomen is a primary location for vata. The body is slightly crooked, with scoliosis, crooked nose, asymmetrical features, or curly hair (the effect of deep movement and hyperactivity in the spine and brain, and mobility). The skin is generally cool to the touch, slightly dry and sometimes stiff (from too much dryness and cold). Brown eyes. Rapid movements, like twitches, or nervous habits like nail biting or foot tapping.

Common complaints: stiffness, especially in joints; fear and anxiety; low back and spinal pain; sciatica; constipation and nervousness. The dryness associated with vata can produce joints that crack with movement. Constipation can be a recurring problem due to excessive peristaltic movements which increase intestinal dryness and inhibit the natural elimination process.

Increasing/decreasing vata: Regardless of constitution, 60% of all ailments are due to an increase in vata because vata controls the mind and most ailments have a mental component. Factors that increase vata are: fear; windy, dry or cold weather; excessive movement; too much mental activity; too much talking, sensory overload; too little water; too much dry food; too much bodily activity. Factors that reduce vata are: meditation; moist heat; heavy foods; slow, non-threatening, manual therapy with warm oil.

Jane came into my office on a cold, windy, dry winter day (factors that can cause vata symptoms in any constitution). I could see immediately that she was anxious. I had her sit next to the heater because warmth counteracts the cold attribute of vata and waited patiently for her to speak, giving space for her nervous system to relax. Almost immediately she began to ramble on and on (nervous rapid speech is a vata trait) about how she was having trouble sleeping, how her low back hurt, and her sciatic pain. I explained the relationship of her problems to the nature of her constitution. She began to relax (understanding her situation quieted the mind and thus sedated the nervous system).

After the initial exchange of information, there was very little verbal interaction between us. The treatment included much manual support and some warm oil, along with gentle micro-movements. Near the end of the session, I had Jane breathe very slowly through the right nostril (a warming breath). I had her move very gently and slowly, then asked her not to move at all but to explore how she felt. The comparison of manageable movement and then stillness offered an inner learning experience that could be built upon. We finished the treatment with some information about things she could do at home to continue to balance her constitution.

THE PITTA (FIRE) CONSTITUTION

The pitta constitution is composed of fire along with a little water. It controls the body's balance of kinetic and potential energies: processes which involve digestion or "cooking" the maturation of food into usable energy or thoughts into theories in the mind. The main fields of activity for pitta are the enzyme and endocrine systems, although pitta is also concentrated in the tissues for digestion of certain substances.

The fire-dominated constitutional type can be very intense, spontaneous, and sometimes a little volatile. When a pitta person is in balance mentally and emotionally, he or she has a great wit and inspiring intelligence, which when unbalanced can turn to a biting, stabbing sarcasm, and egotistical boasting. A pitta type who is in balance may be full of vitality, clear, concise and passionate; we enjoy the vitality and the laughter the pitta inspires. Unbalanced pitta people can be fiery judgmental, aggressive, competitive, hot-tempered, impulsive, rigid and angry most of the time. Physical balance in the pitta is expressed in bright coloring, strong vitality, and balanced structure. When excess pitta is present, the complexion can be red and blemished, the musculature may become excessively tight and constricting, the spine stiff and inflexible.

If the pitta person drinks too much alcohol and/or eats too much spicy food (fuel for the fire), the liver will begin to overwork, the heat rises and tries to get out through the skin, reddening it, the muscles fill with more blood (blood is fire in the human system), the muscles get tense, and hot emotions emerge. The system needs the balancing attributes of cold, moist, and sedative.

When a pitta type sits in the webbed chair, what happens? Heat creates an imprint; think of the broiler marks on a hamburger. If there is an emotional component, usually anger, more heat is produced. What will make the impression stick longest is the pitta tendency to stiffen, which will shut down the fluid action that could flush out the imprint.

Pitta Attributes

Attributes	Manifestations in the Body
Hot	good digestive fire; strong appetite; body temperature tends to be higher than normal; difficulty with heat; loss of hair or baldness; hair slightly oily; tends towards grey hair early in life
Sharp	pointed teeth, penetrating eyes, pointed nose, and chin; heart-shaped face; good absorption and digestion; sharp memory and understanding; tolerant of hard work; irritable
Light	light/medium body frame; does not tolerate bright light; fair shiny skin, bright eyes
Oily	soft oily skin, hair, feces; does not tolerate deep-fried food (irritation in liver and gall bladder)
Liquid	loose liquid stools; hyper-toned muscles; excess urine, sweat and thirst.
Spreading	pitta spreads as rash, acne, inflammation all over the body or on affected areas; pitta subjects want to spread their name and fame all over the country

Pitta body type: medium build, wiry, tight muscles; well-proportioned; penetrating eyes (green, sometimes bloodshot from rising heat in system); sharp features, such as prominent cheek bones or nose. Spine is often very straight and may lack flexibility. Movements are fast and generally precise; when fire is out of control, movements can become reckless. Common complaints: inflammation of joints, tissues, organs. Excess heat can cause problems in liver, blood, gall bladder, and small intestine. As heat rises, migraines, neck and spinal stiffness, fevers, and head congestion can surface. An excess of pitta can produce tension, anger, frustration and bottled-up sadness. Keep in mind that even if you have an air or water constitution, you may develop pitta symptoms.

Increase/decrease in pitta: Factors that increase pitta are: hot foods, alcohol, red meat, too much physical or mental activity, too little liquid, indulgence in anger.

Factors that reduce pitta are: meditation; long slow breathing (especially through left nostril); elongation relaxation of the structure; increasing water in body; opening the heart to softer feelings.

Bob came into my office in the morning after completing his five mile run and drinking three cups of coffee (pitta types are inclined to enjoy coffee, and running gets the pitta revved up). He began to get undressed immediately, ready for action (speed and efficiency and no time to relax are often issues with the fire constitution). I asked, "What would you like to work on?"

In a very loud strong voice (another fire quality) he said, "My body is always tight. I get headaches every afternoon and my neck and chest are stiff." As he spoke he seemed to be getting irritated, and his muscles became tighter around his neck and shoulders.

I asked, "What seems to help when you feel like this?"

"Making love, but that's a problem too because my relationship gets more difficult when I get this uptight. When I make love, and after strenuous exercise, I'm able to relax for a short time, but it doesn't last and I feel worse a few hours later."

In the treatment we spent most of the time exploring subtle work, paying attention to when his "core" seemed to let go, or when he got frustrated with the pacing (the pitta type wants it all right now). I asked him to follow the sense of letting go as it "traveled" throughout the system, and to observe his reactions when nothing was happening. Near the end of the session Bob remarked, "I never knew I could let go without effort, and I never realized how uncomfortable I am when nothing is happening." We ended with some gentle movements he could also do at home to build on the idea of being easy with himself, and some simple breathing exercises to slow the nervous system down so that he could enjoy the space between doing one thing and the next.

THE KAPHA (WATER) CONSTITUTION

Kapha types are composed primarily of the heavy elements of water and earth. The tissues and wastes of the body are the province of kapha. Kapha is the principle of potential energy. There is much stored prana in the heavier elements; to become available for action, fire and air must be added to the water. Consider the person who seems to have so much at their disposal, so much potential, lots of body mass and vitality but it may not be utilized. If only that couch potato could get moving! Kapha controls body stability and lubrication; its basic responsibility is support and protection. Physically, the Kapha person is strong, robust, with great endurance; when unbalanced he is often overweight, congested, and plodding. The predominance of the heavier elements, when in balance, can offer much safety and support. The Kapha person is mentally and emotionally meditative, peaceful, steadfast, sincere, loving, gentle, and tends to have good long-term memory. A kapha type will tend to be dependable, verging on attachment; tender, verging on emotionality due to the watery qualities; fluid in body and mood. When in balance mentally and emotionally, the kapha type is a soothing, calm individual, full of love and compassion; when unbalanced, greed, attachment, and lethargy are common.

When a kapha attribute is increased excessively, such as too much cold moist food (like an ice-cream binge), the heavy wet qualities increase, mobility decreases, the kapha becomes sluggish and congested and may become depressed as his or her energy drops. To come into balance, the kapha would add heat (more pitta) and movement (vata), such as ginger tea and a vigorous walk.

When a kapha type gets up from the webbed chair, he will have deeper dents than the other types because his tissues hold more water, but because of the tendency to flow more readily the imprint will "wash out" quickly. If there is an emotional charge added to the event, like sadness and depression, the combination of body and feeling imprint will stay longer due to the kapha characteristic of attachment.

Kapha Attributes

Attributes	Manifestations in the Body
Heavy	heavy bones, muscles, large body frame; tends to overweight, grounded; deep heavy voice
Slow	slow walk, talk; slow digestion, sluggish metabolism
Cool	cold clammy skin; scanty appetite and thirst; repeated cold, congestion, and cough; desire of hot spicy food
Oily	oily skin, hair and feces; lubricated, unctuous joints and other organs, can tend toward thickness of fluids
Dense	dense pad of fat; thick skin, hair, nail and feces; plump rounded organs
Soft	soft pleasing look; love, care, compassion and kindness
Static	loves sitting, sleeping and doing nothing
Viscous	viscous, sticky, cohesive quality causes compactness, firmness of joints and organs; loves to hug; is deeply attached in love and relationship
Cloudy	in early morning mind becomes cloudy and foggy; often needs coffee stimulant to start the day

Kapha body type: large, heavy, thick, dense, powerful, soft rounded eyes (often blue); movements are slow, steady, plodding, careful.

Common complaints: congestion, overweight, fluid problems, swelling, head colds, lung problems, joint congestion, lethargy, depression and sadness.

Increase/decrease kapha: Factors that increase kapha are: cold foods like dairy products; too much liquid; too much food, especially sweets; sedentary lifestyle; and indulgence in moods.

Factors that reduce kapha are: activity, dry light foods, not too much food, heat either from mild spicy food or from activity that causes sweating.

Willa came into my office complaining of a lack of energy, congestion in the chest and sinuses, and a constant craving for food. As she spoke she began to cry and her body seemed to slump. After the tears subsided, I asked her if she would try an experiment. She nodded. "Could you slowly begin to straighten your spine and lift your head? Notice as you do this what happens inside of you, what you feel."

It took some time but she began to extend herself upward (since the fire element tends to rise, she needed to cultivate both the fire and air in her body to mobilize upward). Her breathing began to get fuller, she got a little more color in her cheeks. As she reached full extension, I asked what she had noticed.

"I feel lighter, and it is easier to breathe." It looked as if she was having a hard time holding the position, so I told her to let herself slowly slump again, noticing how she felt as she did so. She seemed reluctant to give up her new position but soon began to slide downward. When she was in a fully squished position, I asked how she felt.

"Depressed and hungry. I feel the need to be filled up."

"Please try again to elongate." This time it happened almost immediately, and she stayed there with no effort. We continued the treatment both through her movement and some manual intervention. Without being directly challenged to be more active, she embodied the experience that activity can be pleasant and eliminated some of her symptoms. The best healing is experiential learning, in which the nervous system and the entire organism take part.

In the West, we have little or no appreciation for the value of adipose tissues in the organism. Some of our lack of appreciation is due to the cultural self-image we have learned or been taught that an attractive person is one who is slim and athletic. We assume the slender individual is not only more attractive, but healthier and more intelligent. I'm not sure where this idea started, maybe with the advertising industry or from our love affair with the intellect and the body type that generally goes along with it (the intellect is most developed in the pitta person, who also tends to have very little fat). No matter what they do regarding exercise, kapha types generally will have more tissue; no matter how much pitta types may eat, they cannot gain much adipose tissue.

The fact is that adipose tissue is very useful and has many functions in the organism. Healthy meda (adipose tissue) is essential for nourishing the immune system, for maintaining strength, and for proper lubrication of the other layers of tissue. In the building and maintenance of the seven layers of tissue (see Chapter Six), the adipose layer provides nourishment and support for the muscle, blood and plasma. Meda stabilizes the brain and nervous system. In short, if the adipose layer is deficient, many other aspects of the organism are not going to be healthy. We should all have a personal image of wholeness built on a healthy diet, enough exercise, and right thinking, then let the body shape itself around the quality of our attitude and lifestyle.

DETERMINING YOUR CONSTITUTION

With the preceding information and the following chart, try to determine your primary and secondary constitutions. Your primary type is the one you emulate most of the time. The secondary type is one that shows itself under specific conditions, such as mid-summer heat or during extended periods of stress. You may have just enough pitta that when the weather is hot, the heat tips the constitutional scale and you begin to behave as if you were primarily that constitution.

Note: be as honest as you can. Check the description that best defines you from each category. Whenever you find a category where the choice is close between two doshas, check them both. Add up the vata, pitta, and kapha traits. The one with the greatest number will be your main constitutional tendency.

Please remember that a deep understanding of constitution is a fine art developed over many years. This is just to provide a general idea. If you want to investigate your constitution further, locate a qualified Ayurvedic practitioner (see Resources). After determining your constitution, review your type and look carefully at the attributes, which are the secret to maintaining balance.

Constitution Evaluation Chart

	Vata	Pitta	Kapha
Body frame:	thin/frail	muscular/moderate	thick/dense
Body wt.:	light	moderate	heavy
Body ht.:	very tall or short	average	average to tall
Skin:	dry/rough/cold/dark	warm/oily/red	soft/cool/pale
Hair:	dark/curly/dry	blond/red/oily/thin	thick/soft/straight
Eyes:	dark/small	green/bloodshot/penetrating	soft/big/calm
Appetite:	poor/variable	strong	moderate
Thirst:	variable	strong	low
Movement:	excessive	moderate	calm
Sleep:	disturbed	light	deep/excessive
Speech:	excessive	sharp/clear/loud	slow/calm/melodious
Stamina:	tires easily	strong then drops off quickly	enduring
Nails:	brittle/dry/wavy	thin/oily/pointed	flexible/thick/round

RESTORING BALANCE

All the elements are present in every individual, but their proportion and combination vary. Within each person, the balance of the elements may also vary from season to season, or according to time of day. To some degree, health is a result of keeping our individual qualitative and quantitative balance of the five elements.

When the proportions are upset, disease may result. Increased earth can result in obesity, increased water can lead to edema, increased fire can cause fever and ulcers. Changes in the mental faculties may appear when the equilibrium is upset, such as aggravated air causing fear and anxiety, fire leading to anger and hate, earth bringing depression and dullness.

The elements of life are constantly in motion. The elements that predominate in us at any given time represent what we need to work on. Once we understand the elemental patterns, we can learn to use them to our benefit. There are very few people who are so strongly dominated by a particular element that balance cannot be restored.

Looking again at the impression made by the chair with the waffle pattern, we see someone with a watery kapha constitution, or maybe someone who just ate ice cream during lunch (a cold sweet food that increases congestion and stagnation in the body) took a nap in the chair, which increased stagnation and compression of the tissues. (Sweet taste, cold, liquid, stagnation, and so on increase kapha.) When this person awoke, it took great effort to get out of the chair because he felt heavy (another attribute) and a little low energetically. When another person laughed at the pattern on his legs, he got embarrassed and depressed (a kapha emotional attribute), and since the emotion of depression tends to be heavy, it added to the physical pattern.

How do we avoid or reduce the imprint? When we first notice that the seat of the chair has a waffle pattern, we should suspect that part of us will sooner or later begin to sink into it. Awareness is always the key to change. We can stop the action right then and there by getting a cushion for the chair or by choosing another seat. If the impression is already established, we can increase movement (vata) in the tissues, creating friction (a little pitta heat) by moving around a bit. Or we can take action by rubbing the back of the legs vigorously, increasing the circulation, moving fluids, and increasing the heat and movement manually.

There are also other ways to use this constitutional information. For example, the next time you are taking some medicine, food, or food supplement, make an effort to find out the attributes of the substance. What is the proposed action of the substance? What elements would it represent? For instance, you have a dull aching headache (dull pain is a kapha type of pain) and take an aspirin. Aspirin is sour, which increases pitta (fire) and thus would increase circulation, an appropriate action for your kapha headache. As you prepare to swallow the pills, imagine their action before they enter your system by visualizing (vata) the increased circulation breaking up the congestion in the head. The actions of most common substances are available in other Ayurvedic texts, or your health practitioner will know the actions of the substances that are being prescribed. With this information, you can become an active participant in the healing process.

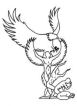

Chapter Three

Changing the Self-Image

Everyone should learn to analyze themselves dispassionately...
Find out what you are, not what you imagine you are!

\- Paramahansa Yogananda

Imagine going back to a time before you were born, before you had a body or any connection to the desires and needs that stem from having a body. Imagine you are free from thought and emotions. You are pure consciousness, at one with God. Imagine residing in a heavenly state of peace, or visualize a peaceful resting place beside a springtime brook.

After an indeterminate time, you hear God call: "Have I got a job for you!" Or, looking at it another way, a memory of "unfinished business" arises and your karma of leftover tasks and desires calls to you. This summons stimulates your thought forms (composed of air and ether) and brings on more memories. You get excited, which can be construed as nerve energy, and are no longer as restful. From a state of pure spirit, you begin to spiral downward into denser matter.

You choose your parents and conception occurs. You are no longer as spacious as you once were. Although you have not yet identified yourself with this developing body, it becomes more dominant as cells multiply, a brain and spinal cord develop. This embryo is already much heavier than the thoughts that created it.

You take birth in the physical world and now you are much more restricted. Soon you start to build a self-image around this heavy ele-

mental form because of its constant need for food, air, and elimination. Bodily chemistry is cumbersome compared to the being of pure spirit you were. You begin to connect to events outside of yourself and start to identify yourself as this vehicle, as something other than spirit. Consider the implications.

THE INTERNAL AND EXTERNAL ENVIRONMENTS

Once we are contained in the physical form, we interact with two distinct environments: the outer and inner. The internal environment pertains primarily to spirit, to the deep place within us, the vantage point from which we can observe the drama of life. To experience ourselves as something other than the whole existence of the cosmos from which we came, we have to identify ourselves as a separate unit of matter: "Me" rather than "the One." This process starts with the first cell or group of cells which are encased in membranes.

The next physical development is the growth of the spine and brain. In Ayurveda, the cerebral-spinal fluid is called the shushumna, the "spiritual waters" the material that is closest to pure light or pure consciousness in human beings. Imagine this essential liquid circulating through your very core, around your brain and through a tube-like structure in the center of your spine, widening and narrowing rhythmically like the wave action on the ocean. Both Eastern and Western sages tell us to "Seek the kingdom of God within." The spinal tube and its contents are the physical representation of the personal inner kingdom. Here you can rest; here you can be close to spirit.

As we continue to grow and encase our developing parts with more membranes, the light of awareness, the consciousness of who we are, continues to be present within every cell.

The inside environment is a safe house. It is a place we can return to whenever we need rest and renewal. During times of intense pain, we naturally retreat there. If we can go deep enough and settle ourselves in that place through a great night's sleep, a deep meditation, or even a coma state in traumatic situations when we come "back out" we're refreshed, ready to face the battles of the world. We cannot stay just in our inner environment, but we can regularly immerse ourselves deeply enough within so we can carry that inner peace into our actions in the world.

The external environment is the place where we share with others and where we can have an effect on the planet. It is also a place of constant change; we can't depend on it for safety and support. The elements change their nature continuously, modified by temperature, humidity, time and seasons. We know, for instance, that the weather won't be constant from season to season or even hour to hour. We are also constantly changing cells are growing and dying, thoughts are coming and going, hair is graying and falling out, everything in the outside environment is always in flux. This is true for our family environment, work environment, community and society.

The "land of enchantment" outside ourselves seems to have so much to offer. "Oh, that's a nice person. She gives me something to eat when I'm hungry and makes those little kootchy-kootchy koo noises. I miss that person when she's not here." I've created a major attachment to the outside world and am becoming dependent on externals. If I don't have food, I start to feel uncomfortable. If I don't get a little of that kootchy-kootchy-koo once in a while, I start to feel sad.

Ladies and gentlemen, step right up to the center ring in the circus of life. The "greatest show on earth" is the external environment where we get so involved with experiences, events, things and people that our internal spiritual selves get overshadowed. As our nervous systems develop, our awareness becomes less focused on who we are and turns more to how we entertain ourselves. We begin to be so enchanted by the many external distractions that we are slowly drawn away from our real home within. Eventually we may come to believe the bodily form is who we are. At some point in life, most of us have so much going on in the outer environment that we forget where we came from and how to get back in. We're stuck in the land of enchantment.

I'm not saying this is wrong. I'd rather think of this predicament as educational; there is something to be learned here and shared with others who are as trapped as we are. Some people look upon this world as illusory, as maya. It's not that illusory if you get hit by a truck, right? Most of us awaken each day stuck in our bodies and proceed with the daily grind, but if we become more flexible, we have the option of looking at our situation another way: "Wow, what can I learn today? How can I share who I really am in here with that person who's walking down the street in such a bad mood? How can I remind him, through my actions or words, of who he really is?"

In other words, how can we awaken to the reality of our spiritual selves and return from the land of enchantment? Not being great sages, perhaps, but simply compassionate souls, can we help awaken others? In my experience in the field of bodywork and personal development with many clients over the last twenty-five years, I have observed that when we loosen the historic imprints of body and mind, then the inner knowledge of who we really are can begin to shine forth again. The point is not to become disenchanted with the outer world, but to become enchanted with our inner and outer life and all the movement that takes place between the two environments.

SELF-IMAGE

We start our journey through life free from any agenda. From this place of spontaneity and curiosity, we start building a self-image based, on the one hand, on useful and changeable ideas about ourselves, and on the other hand, on assumptions, habits, and internal and external pressures. As soon as we move from our home base in spirit, we establish separation and a different sort of self-identification, one related to approval by the outside environment, such as approval from our parents.

There we are lying in our crib, contentedly playing with our toes and getting used to this bodily container, when Mother enters the room and draws our attention outward into the external environment. "Oh, I need a nice hug from that person..." An attachment is building to the outside environment. We are beginning to develop a different idea of who we are relative to Mom. Now we are her "sweet little thing," or her "little cutie." Any number of images builds our self-image. As time passes, we might become "you little brat" or "the one who never listens." The more we identify with this outside world, the more we assume these identities and subsequently shape our tissues in a way that represents these ideas.

As life goes on, we are influenced by a wider range of pressures from society, peers, teachers, bosses any number of sources that demand our attention. It is focused awareness that etches the flesh, freezing it into the pattern that tells us who we are, or at least who we have become. Through consciousness and the five elements, we create and shape our self-image, adding our beliefs, habits and experiences. As habits and beliefs become hardened, the nervous system gets patterned and anchors in the physical body through the bones and membranes. As we harden around our developing identities, the heavier elements create the "hard copy" and we develop an agenda, reinforcing this by choosing an environment that is supportive of our beliefs, friends who think as we do, familiar events, qualities, even foods. Seeing is believing. Our surroundings and behavior reflect back to us just who we think we are, building more and more proof to sustain the limitations that identity requires.

In World War I, the soldiers had defective helmets which left parts of the back of the neck uncovered. Bullets and shrapnel, small bits of metal from bombs, would sometimes get lodged in the back of the soldiers' heads where the eye nerves are located. When their progress was followed, it was found that a great percentage of the surviving soldiers went through a similar process at home: withdrawing from their families and not being able to communicate. They would start to stumble, to miss things they reached for, and then they would go into a very deep depression and sometimes die.

A young physician, sitting with one of these injured soldiers, reached out and silently offered him a cigarette. There was no response. After some time of extending the offered cigarette, the physician started to get angry and said, "Do you want this or not?" At the sound of the physician's voice, the soldier shifted his perspective and reached out and took the cigarette. The physician started to wonder if the soldier had seen him at first, and, after examination, he realized that the soldier's field of vision had narrowed to such a degree that he was, to all purposes, almost blind. As a result of this new information, the doctors had the injured soldiers wear dark glasses so they would have to reach out with different senses. The soldiers started behaving more normally in dealing with their impairment. Their eyes didn't get better, but the depression and the loss of contact with the world went away.

The soldiers' visual range had been getting so small that they were losing touch with life; they were narrowing their focus without knowing it. The soldiers had a physical limitation which was creating their impression of life. Like the soldiers, we must participate in our own healing by learning about our condition so we can upgrade our images of ourselves. To do so we must use introspection and, on occasion, have someone else to hold up the mirror, whether that be a therapist, partner, child, or the deep reflection of our inner vision.

If we rely primarily on one sense or one attitude, or our history of belief, like the soldier we will be missing the greater picture of life around us. If we become completely accustomed to our own view to the exclusion of all others, our feelings and beliefs get etched into the patterns of our brain and tissues. To be able to change, we need to shift our perspective and move into a place where the brain and nervous system can observe dispassionately, where we can sit while we take inventory and reevaluate our actions, feelings, and beliefs.

Before we can activate change, we have to stop our dance with the land of enchantment long enough to see who we are and what we are doing. As long as the car engine is running and we are in motion, that which we can perceive out the car window is limited to that which we glimpse quickly in passing. We may get the general lay of the land, but fail to notice particulars, such as the sign indicating the bridge up ahead is out. This dynamic is also true in our organism: if we are always in motion, filling each moment with thoughts and actions, it is impossible to observe ourselves and evaluate the need for change. Another possibility is that those of us with a kapha-type constitution may be moving at such a leisurely pace that we get lulled into complacency, missing the signals for change in that way. To evaluate our self-image, we must be able to change our rhythm, shift gears. When we slow down our vehicle, we can take more in visually. When we turn the engine off, we can feel the wind blow, hear the birds sing, smell the flowers in the air.

Have you ever gotten so busy that you forgot to eat? Probably not if you are a kapha or pitta, but if you are a vata person with that wonderfully active mind and rapidly moving nervous system, you may often forget. If you are a kapha type, you may not recognize your need for exercise. You get so cozy, so laid back and satisfied just sitting on the couch, that your metabolism and heart rate are not important. If you are a pitta, with your great intelligence, high energy, and strong will, you may not notice your emotional needs. To become aware of our personal need for change, we must first stop our habitual acts so we get another perspective on ourselves. How do we slow our engine, shift attention effectively to a point where we can view our action/inaction, our beliefs, our general state of being? We want to move into a dispassionate place of observation so we can see what we need, and then find out how to act on that information.

Resting in Neutral

If we want to change directions in our automobile, we must stop for a moment, come into a place of non-doing, or neutral. As long as the car is in gear, we can't reverse our direction. Even to make a turn we must downshift, a momentary break in the functioning of the vehicle. The same is true of our bodies and minds. For the nervous system to make a new choice, to change course, there must be a momentary pause. The pause in action is what I call resting in neutral. If we want to improve our ability to make choices, to function more efficiently, and to learn from our experiences, we need to be able to rest in neutral.

As we move from inner to outer environments, or bring thought into action, it is wise to have a moment of rest in neutral so we might have time to reconsider, adjust slightly, or even to change our intent completely if need be. Physically, the place where we can rest in neutral is the space between the layers of membranes, a space in the synapse of the nerves; in short, a space that we make available and utilize. To do this we must be aware of the fact that we have this space, adequate vata, and sufficient support for the time out. If our tissues are compressed with historic events and our functional capacity is "reading" a lack of space, we are going to act in a hasty fashion for fear of not having the support we need. Did you ever find yourself on the verge of losing your balance while holding something delicate in your hand, like a cup of hot tea? You hurry to put it down and wind up spilling tea all over the place. This is the same as the internal experience when we have no place to rest in neutral, no place to store information about having a choice.

After the fact we often think "If I had only said this," or "I should not have said that," or "I should have turned left, then I never would have gotten into this mess." More intelligent choices were available to us, but we weren't able to stop long enough in neutral to hear the right choice come from the internal environment, that place of rest and peace. We need to bring that place actively back into our daily lives. One way to access the neutral space in our lives, both in thought and action, is to acknowledge first of all that there is a neutral, and appreciate the time between doing one thing and the next.

In our busy Western society, we think of down time as wasted time, nobody's making money or getting things done, nobody's producing the product. In India, and in some other countries in which I've traveled, the people appreciate the so-called "non-doing" time. I was in New Delhi about a month or so after I arrived in India when some new arrivals joined our group. They said, "Come with us to the bank, it will only take a little while."

"I'll take a book." I already knew these transactions don't happen quickly in India.

One lady said, "Don't bother. All I'm going to do is change a traveler's check."

I took the book anyway. After they'd been in line for hours, the new arrivals were emanating that old Western "come on and hurry up" energy. The bank personnel were getting irritated with their impatience, so the Indians took a tea break. Have you noticed when you are most in a hurry is when things really slow down? Obstacles get in the way, the traffic increases. Meanwhile, the bank personnel noticed I was out in front of the bank patiently reading my book. The next thing I knew, the guard had brought me a cup of chai (Indian tea) and was telling me about his family; we discussed the best places to go in town, how not to get overcharged, and so on. I was resting in neutral and the energy from that place attracted attention. Meanwhile my friends were emotionally upset, tense, and had symptoms like tight muscles and headaches.

The great sages and yogis say live in the moment, there we will find the answers and the peace we seek. One way to enjoy a moment-to-moment lifestyle is to rest in neutral, and one way to do that is to get physically in touch with the membrane layers of our bodies where we may be historically laminated, release the membrane hardening, and reclaim the area.

What if you closed your eyes right now and put all your attention on your breath? Can you find where your breath starts? Is it in your chest, your belly, or somewhere else? As the breath moves in your body, can you feel the ribs moving? How about the spine, does it move when you breathe? Can you feel your diaphragm moving down as you inhale? If you stop to notice any of these things, you will surely change in some meaningful way because you will have rested in neutral and reclaimed your space within the membrane layers.

Going back to the analogy of a car, we have to shift into neutral before getting into reverse. We have to shift into neutral before going into a higher gear. If we want to go faster, we have to go, at least momentarily, to a neutral place or we'll strip our gears or rupture our disks or pull our shoulders out. If we free ourselves to move through the membrane boundaries at will, make the membranes semi-permeable by using the elements and our attention, have no emotional resistance and a clear sense neurologically of how to get there, we can rest in neutral. This sounds like a tall order, but we already know how to do most of those things. We just need to take the time, get into ourselves, and go for the ride.

Exercise:

In the following exercise, awareness will increase through touch. Pay particular attention to stopping. It is that resting place which must be acknowledged.

Resting in Neutral

Either you or your partner lie on your back. Bring the knees up to soften the underlying tissues and relax the navel. You may want to put a pillow underneath your knees and provide support under the right elbow of the active person. Remember, increasing support and safety encourages positive change.

Close your eyes. Take a moment to consider your navel. At one point in our development, we got all our nourishment and connection to the world through our navel. Our membranes developed from blood circulating through the navel connection to our mothers, our lifeline to the physical world. There are still vestigial connections, leftover layers of tissue, from the navel to every portion of our bodies, however dried up from disuse or folded over or twisted they may be.

Bring all the fingers and thumb of your right hand, (if you have a partner they take over from here) together to a single point. Rest the fingers gently around the navel. It is essential to take a moment of rest here; it's the point of the whole exercise. You are resting in neutral (both parties.) Nothing particular is happening in your mind.

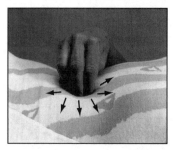 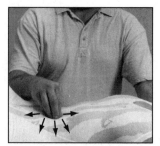

Subtly begin exploring any direction in which the navel would like to move. Very slowly move it only 1/16th of an inch in any direction. Slide it left or right, up or down, to the corners. Move in the direction that seems easiest, but stop completely after each movement and wait for the awareness to gather.

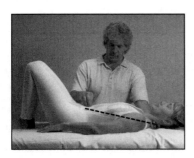 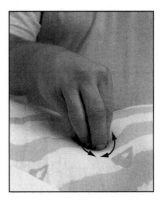

When the ease of movement seems to slow down or stop, hold at that place. This is now neutral. After stopping for a moment, then exaggerate the movement very slightly in that same direction. Take it just a little farther, then stop again. This action increases the awareness in mind, body and energy. Awareness, safety and support are the three keys to making positive change.

Notice what happens when you exaggerate. Does something change under the fingers or deeper? Does the breath change, the back soften? See if something else is transpiring. Come back to the original "neutral." Explore another directional drift from here, and follow that movement.

With your hand still slightly exaggerating one of the directions, can you feel a connection to some part of you farther up in your body from where the movement is happening? Breathe from the other end of the connection several times, using your breath to make it stronger.

Stop and rest your arm. You are now in a new neutral place with yourself. Enjoy. You may complete more directions if you choose, but don't overdo it. Stop after one or two more, notice differences, then go about your normal activities.

You're Okay, I'm Okay

Mostly we describe ourselves to someone else by telling something about ourselves, which is not truly who we are inside. Who are we in the world, when we meet the boss, when we see our children? Who are we are on a "good day" or a "bad day?" Wearing different masks and attitudes to fit each different scene, we get confused as to our identity. If we wear a particular attitude regularly enough, we begin to think that is who we are. It is only when we seek the essence behind the masks that we progress toward becoming happy.

The physical form reflects back to us our ideas of who we are, a stronger more visible image of what has been conceived in the idea form and we get programmed by its reflection. We must be able to shed superficial beliefs, such as "I am a person who has a mustache, is about 6 feet tall and slightly overweight." We have such a strong identification with our physical form: the "hard copy" of who we think we are, the printout of our inner beliefs and attitudes. If we can melt away the historic imprints held in the flesh, the ideas that held them in place also can be updated, and we can slowly peel away the layers and return to ourselves.

One of the most liberating ideas we may entertain is that we are perfect just the way we are and that our "good" and "bad" traits are all in place precisely to further our personal growth. That may be true, yet we always seem to be striving to rid ourselves of the "bad" habits of nagging or anger, or the bad back that prevents us from being more physically active. Poor digestion may inspire us to fast, to start a spring cleaning of the body, to eat new foods and do yoga, but so often these tend to be temporary measures and we soon find ourselves stuck back in the same old "bad" habits.

Imagine yourself as a pitta person who is interested in being more receptive. Maybe a relationship has failed due to lack of receptivity, or some other interpersonal encounter ended on a bad note for the same reason. You begin with the resolve, "I'm going to be more receptive, listen before I speak, get all the information before I respond." As a fire person, you have the tendency to be impulsive, even explosive; it's in the nature of the elements and undoubtedly in your self-image. Maybe the resolve can be maintained for a while because the pitta person has a strong will, but soon things break down again.

The next step becomes, "I'll get some counseling." Therapy goes well, unearthing many remembrances of how you were never given a chance to respond as a child. "I understand; surely I can now be more receptive." Each time the inclination comes up to tell someone else how it really is, you remember your childhood self and hold your tongue. But deep inside, you are getting angry. It doesn't fit your self-image to be so subservient, so you have a few beers, which heats up your liver and increases the fire. You get up in the morning and run five miles, which heats your entire system. Your muscles get tight, your attitude gets tight, and you are ripe to tell off the next person who speaks to you, a return to the old habit.

How do you see yourself at this moment? Looking at myself, I would say that I'm a tall, middle-aged teacher and bodyworker. Maybe in a different context, I might say, "I'm a shy, quiet person." There are any number of other ways to describe myself, but each description sets up limitation, and as soon as I establish certain things about myself, I have re-enforced my own limitations. For example, I don't dance, something that I've wanted to change for years. Earlier in my life, friends would encourage me to get out there and dance, which only made me more self-conscious and more inhibited. At this point most people don't encourage me to dance any more because they know it probably won't work and I'll be uncomfortable. Now they see me as I do, a non-dancer. My personal self-image is being supported by my group of friends. After some time holding that impression or image, the body shapes around the belief. I used to try to dance when no one was around imagining myself dancing at a party when the music was playing. As the years and the image have had more time to "set up," I rarely imagine myself as a dancer even when alone.

Did you ever notice how a person exhibits in their physical form some indication of their actions, occupation, and "stance" in life? Look at a football player. Even without the uniform, you can tell by the shape and organization of his body that the nature of the person's activity is clearly athletic and prepared for action. Can you imagine his self-image being anything other than "ready for action," with every sense, nerve, and muscle primed for the next play? The athlete must have that self-image to be at the top of his game. But what about when the uniform comes off? Can he take a different stance in life, can the image be shifted?

A number of years ago, Mr. M, a blind man, was curious about the many different healing arts, so he decided to take a year-long sabbatical, travel around and find whomever he could to assist him in whatever ways they might. He ended up coming to me on one of the last legs of his trip.

"So what have you learned on your journey?"

He said, "Well, this person said that my head was too far

back and that's why I was getting neck pains and stressing my shoulder."

I said, "Okay. What else?"

"This other person said that my right shoulder is much too far forward and stiff, that I don't allow that shoulder to be flexible and that, too, creates a problem in my neck and back."

"Structurally speaking, that's reasonable."

"Somebody else said that my chest was too far forward and that put a strain in my mid-back."

"Okay. That's interesting." I could see each time he said something, he was starting to feel a little heavier. I said, "Well, before we start working, let me say a few things here. I assume, not knowing much about being blind, that you may run into things from time to time. If I were you, I'd put my chest right out front so I'd bang into my chest before I'd bang into my face, which means I'd pull my head back."

He started to lighten up a little bit. I said, "I notice you use cane techniques, and the best way to do that is to get your shoulder out there so you can work with your cane. Makes sense to me. That's perfect. You know, the last thing in the world you'd want to bang into is your head."

By that time, tears were coming down his face. He said, "Geez, maybe I'm okay the way I am. But I have pain."

I said, "We've established that how you are is very important much of the time. But you also understand by your pain that if you stay that way all the time, it does create problems. First accept exactly how you are and know that that's okay when you're moving around in the world and in an environment you're not used to. But when you're home and you're comfortable and you know where things are, let it go, relax and release the pattern of strain."

Mr. M had a chance to review his image of himself and

accept it. With this in place, the work to make improvements was much easier. We undertook some hands-on work and movement techniques to release the historic automatic patterning. We had found the relationship of when he needed the protective pattern of his body and when he did not, and only then did we work with a system whereby he could "take off" the pattern when he was in a safe familiar environment. The essence of the treatment was to give validation, options, functional release, and something to grow on, all in relationship to the self-image.

We all have our blind spots, don't we? Put yourself in the position of one who was blind from birth. "I wonder what I look like to others in the world? Am I okay, do I look funny?" Can you imagine developing a self-image with no visual reference? So much of our self-image is built around our assumptions relative to others and our outside environment. It is a profound experience to ponder the idea that we are okay just the way we are.

YOU ARE OKAY THE WAY YOU ARE

SAFETY AND SUPPORT

Even though it is important to accept ourselves as we are, we still want to be able to change whatever doesn't work very well any more, to make ourselves flexible enough to access our own inner wisdom, to become more fully "who we are." The body is an effective tool for change primarily because it is honest in its expression. The mind can give excuses, create new beliefs to cover what is not comfortable; we may be denying our emotions, but we can use the body to evaluate the nervous system, to feed new information to the brain, and to elicit material from emotional storage.

All too often we are rudely awakened to our need for change by that age-old teacher pain in the physical body. Usually, we don't see any reason to change unless discomfort arises in our life. However, we actually have an equal opportunity to awaken through an increase in bodily comfort or pleasure, or just curiosity about something new. Generally speaking, a subtle increase or decrease in comfort or pleasure can inspire positive change; big changes are often too much for the general patterns of the system and may even cause a recoil. Therefore, to elicit change we must uncover our needs with awareness, safety, and support.

So where do we get these attributes of safety, support, and awareness? Deep within us we have a memory of safety. After all, we are connected with spirit or God; how much safer can we get? But after taking birth and encasing the spirit in flesh the need to eat and sleep, likes and dislikes, sensory stimuli, our attachments, we begin to forget and feel separated from that source of safety and support. What do we do while we are adrift, until we are safe at home again in spirit?

First we have to understand how we separate ourselves from our habitual patterns, which can be accomplished through deep introspection and by looking at ourselves from different perspectives. When we only see ourselves from our current point of view composed of our historic imprints and beliefs and habits we lose perspective. For example, by viewing ourselves only through the Western scientific model, we lose sight of our more non-linear side. If we look solely at the esoteric side, we don't take the necessary concrete steps to make changes. In order to utilize our true self in our life, take positive action, and be more free to enjoy life, we need awareness of our entire makeup, such as an understanding of the elements and the way we function on a bio-mechanical level, as well as more clarity about our mental and emotional patterns. Once we get enough information or awareness, we can peel away the veils of illusion and create more safety and support.

As we use our bodies in the world, strong influences from the outside environment can cause dysfunction, or even the complete destruction of the system. This is why we need the inner environment as a safe place, a place of relative peace. The more we go external to ourselves, the greater the question of safety. How thick do I need my boundaries if I'm going to carry a big sack of nails on my shoulder every day? It's going to be thicker up here, right? How big do I need my abdomen to be if I'm going to work with people's emotional stuff all day? I'll thicken up a bit. We embody a lot of thought and a lot of purpose, not just bio-mechanical actions.

The ability to change is a direct result of the safety we feel within and around us at all times. Some years ago I studied a psychotherapy process called Hakomi therapy. Hakomi is an American Indian word that means: How do I stand in relation to these many worlds? To me this translates as: Who am I in relation to my environments? Who am I both inside and out? There are many methods for getting in tune with the presence of spirit within, an essential step in recognizing the support and safety we have within us at all times. But how do we deal with unsafe situations?

Mrs. G. was given a hysterectomy. She had a natural tendency to avoid the lower abdomen, to move around the area rather than through it. She said it seemed numb and distant to her. Even her legs and lower back seemed less available for support. Her history prior to the surgery included many years of chronic infections, pain and discomfort in the low abdomen and pelvis, cysts on the ovaries, and prior to these problems she had been sexually molested as a child. Why would anyone want to inhabit a place with that kind of history?

We started with the feet and lower legs, freeing the holding pattern in that area. Then I had her sit up and put weight on one foot at a time while I placed my hands on her spine in various places. She was to tell me when she felt the pressure (which she was creating with her foot) arrive at my hands. When she felt the vertebra move, she would sigh in relief.

Later, we worked with her chest and upper back in order to free her breathing. I asked, "How far down can you feel the breath?" Slowly, with each breath, it got lower, until finally she could feel her pelvis. In this way, we used areas which were safe to introduce awareness and support from her own body until she could include the previously unsafe abdominal area into her self-image. When it's safe, we can investigate and make choices. Mrs. G first had the opportunity to realize: "Wow, I've got legs; I have a nice housing of rib cage; I have oblique muscles; I have a pelvic floor. I actually have a lot of support."

To change the self-image, one must have adequate support and safety and a generous helping of personal awareness. If it's not safe enough to make a change, why bother? It doesn't matter if your peer group or your lover or your friends all say you should have a long-term relationship; if that's not safe for you, there's no way it will happen. Before we get involved with bio-chemical and bio-mechanical changes, before psychological introspection or re-balancing the elements of our constitution, we must have awareness, safety and support. With these qualities in place, all changes are possible.

Positive changes are first preceded by new awareness the spiritual aspect within us all that must be addressed in order to accomplish change. No matter which method is used or even with the assistance of a practitioner, awareness is the true healer, awareness of being one with spirit, awareness of our wholeness and awareness of our ability to improve. We can change our self-image by expanding our view of ourselves. We can scrutinize our behavior, actions, and habits closely, with a great amount of attention. If necessary, with enough safety and support, we can go back the same way we came, retrace our actions, behaviors and habits to their source. We have to be able to shift our vantage point and stop the automatic action or behavior, then we can settle back into our inner environment, rest in neutral, and from there emerge with whatever action is needed.

A pitta constitutional tendency is to think that more is better, as in doing more because it feels good. This tends to overload the system with actions, essentially shutting down the ability to observe intelligently and to clarify specific needs. A vata type may conclude that he just needs to think things through, his usual modus operandi, to find his need for change, with a typical outcome of more confusion and less clarity. Because vata is responsible for 60% of all disease, we all use this excuse. Then there is the kapha strategy of it's all going to be okay, go with the flow. The problem is that nothing gets done and the person does not change.

The task of clarifying who we are could start with updating the most evident representation of who we have become, which is contained in the physical form. What is needed is to create a more permeable, flexible, physical form that can reflect who we are inside at our deepest core, and at the same time have the pliability to respond to our outer environment and shape itself around our daily tasks in life. Some of who we are may not be accessible to change. For example, our constitution stays the same throughout our lives. It is something we must adjust to, learn what to do in order to stay in relative balance.

If we review the attributes of each element and their rela-tionship to our constitution, we can begin to put together some idea of which elements need to be augmented or reduced in order to increase our level of awareness, support and safety to regain or sustain balance. The key to simple use of the Ayurvedic information is understanding the attributes; how they affect us and our personal relationship to life. By choosing foods and activities that enhance or reduce the attributes of the elements, affect our thinking, and govern our energy flow, we can build more support and safety into our very makeup. By using the information from the last chapter to understand our attributes and by exploring some of the following exercises, we may increase our ability to see ourselves from different per-spectives.

The brain and the nervous system learn by comparing differences.
-Moshe Feldenkrais

Before trying the following exercises, you may want to review the section on determining constitution. Or you can simply try all three methods and see what works, what increas-es your feeling of personal safety and security.

Exercise:
Bringing Balance to Your Constitution

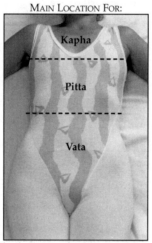

MAIN LOCATION FOR:

The three areas of constitutional focus

The vata person, when out of balance, has the following attributes: very active mind, nervousness, anxiety, and tends to be cold and dry.

Prepare a hot water bottle, some warm oil, a fresh towel, and a blanket.

Lie on the back and notice what parts of your body are relaxed and what parts are not; your thoughts; and your level of safety. Apply warm oil to the low abdomen, from the pelvic bones to the navel, cover with the towel, and place hot water bottle on top of towel. Place the blanket over the whole body, with a pillow under the knees. The warm oil reduces the dryness and warms the body; the blanket offers security.

Place hands on the lower abdomen (the location of the downward directional energy) and slowly breathe in, feeling the abdomen rise and fall with each breath. Feel you are absorbing the heat and unctuousness of the oil. Do this for several minutes, then rest.

Place the hands very lightly on the sides of the head, just above the ears (this is where the cranial fluid movement is most easily felt). Feel the subtle movements of widening and narrowing under your hands. Let your breath come naturally. Continue for as long as comfortable.

Observe again your level of comfort, safety, and relaxation. Follow this exercise with a cup of hot mild ginger tea with cream and honey (this increases the digestive strength and warms the system).

The pitta person, based on his main attributes, may have too much heat in the system, be overly intellectual, have hypertoned tissues, and volatile emotions. These are the troublesome qualities of an imbalance, and we all may have some of these.

Preparation: Soak two cotton balls in cold milk, soak a towel in cold water and wring it out.

Lie on your back. Notice if there are areas of your body that are tense and are not resting on the surface support. Compare your two sides for differences. Note the spinal muscles and tone of the abdomen.

Place the cotton balls on closed eyelids. Feel the cool sensation rush through the eyes and head. Draw in a long slow breath, either through the left nostril while closing off the right, or by rolling your tongue into a tube and breathing in through the mouth. Both these methods cool the system. Do this several times.

Very lightly tense the entire body from the head down to

the toes, then release with a gentle sigh. Do this three times, then relax entirely. This releases the areas that are tight.

Place the cold towel on the abdomen, covering the area between the diaphragm and the navel. Breathe in the same way you did before, imagining the coolness entering the liver and gallbladder. On the exhalation, think about the heart softening and the energy of the heart expanding. The energy centered in the heart is in charge of dispersal; let it disperse the heat of the pitta region. Keep your attention on the area of the heart and rest as long as you feel comfortable, noting differences from when you first began.

The kapha constitution is often hindered in the attempt to maintain balance or change the self-image by the attributes of stagnation, coldness, attachment, lethargy, slowness, and moodiness.

Lie on your back and notice your level of energy. From the diaphragm, begin short rapid breathing, like a bellows blowing on the embers of a fire (this enhances internal fire, adding heat to the cold constitution). Do this for a few minutes, then check your energy level.

Go for a walk or walk in place for ten minutes, breathing deeply (movement breaks up stagnation and congestion, and reduces lethargy). Note your attitude. Movement will often make you feel lighter in spirit. (Breathing from the diaphragm and movement increase the upward directed vital air.)

Lie on your back again. Notice your energy level and the feeling you have about life.

The types of responses vary from constitution to constitution. For example, if you have much water and earth in your system (kapha constitution), you already have the support which is a natural attribute of these heavy elements. Increasing safety and support may permit you to be more open to certain lessons in life. The downside of an abundance of kapha is that awareness, which circulates in the system through the elements of air and ether, can get congested and you may not be able to perceive clearly the dangers about you, or the subtleties of a situation. Thus the work of a kapha might be to keep the water element under control by increasing body movement and the kinesthetic sense.

The rest of this book offers some concrete ideas of how we can understand what separates us from our safety, both internally and externally, and how we can change our relationship to our own boundaries by melting away the life impressions that are no longer supportive.

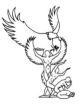

Chapter Four

Membrane Function: Safety and Support

Be calmly active and actively calm.

- Paramahansa Yogananda

WHAT ARE MEMBRANES?

After many years of practice in the field of somatic therapy, I was asked to sit in on a chiropractic medical dissection, in trade for teaching some chiropractic students. Day by day, the instructor removed various body parts from the cadaver and explained their importance: "This is the brachial plexus nerve, and this and that are what it does... this is the biceps muscle, the femur, the frontal bone..." By my third visit, the cadaver had been disassembled quite completely, leaving only a deflated sack of skin and membranes. One student in the back said, "Doctor, what is that stuff remaining on the table?" The doctor dismissed the leftovers with a wave of his hand. "Those are just the connective tissue membranes that held the parts in place."

The doctor was coming from a system that valued the separate components more than the membranes that held them in place and in relationship to each other but, to me, all the "important" body parts had no functional potential whatsoever in a living body without being contained in boundaries and connected to each other. It was like having a pile of expensive computer components not hooked up with each other.

To maintain our individual space and our bodily integrity, we must contain ourselves, assume some degree of separation person-to-person, environment-to-environment, and body part-to-body part. Expanding outward from the center of the body, the membranes are utilized to separate our inside from the outside, the right from the left, what's me and mine from what is something or somebody else's. What's me and what's the floor? Is this my pain or yours? If we don't have boundaries, things get very confusing, if not dangerous. We may merge too much with others. We may confuse our ideas about who we are with those of our families or occupations and forget the real self the one connected to spirit. Because of the way we've been taught to visualize ourselves, we have defined ourselves as separate parts, as separate beings. This is exaggerated in any educational process that tends to teach things in parts, as the doctor was doing in his dissection, and not emphasize or value interrelationship.

As opposed to the Western model, the Ayurvedic system begins with a study of the interrelationship of the whole and later breaks down into a study of the separate parts. Imagine some of the many layers within us: the membranes that wrap the bones of the spine, the membranes that surround the muscles next to the spine, the membranes around the ribs, the epidermal and dermal layers of skin. To regain or develop a sense of our wholeness, we must understand how the membranes maintain us as separate parts and how those parts are related; we must see the membranes as containers, not as barriers. We need to have enough awareness of and interaction with our membranes so we can move through the boundaries at will, outward from the inside environment and inward from the outside environment.

Let's say we're on a small side road traveling from Arizona

to New Mexico. "This is nice countryside here," you say. "I wonder if we're still in Arizona?" Short of seeing a border sign, you don't know. The earth doesn't distinguish between this land over here as Arizona and over that line there as New Mexico. Rather than having an image of ourselves as whole beings, we tend to envision our bodies as full of border signs. The mind has been trained to think that the finger stops here, and then there's the palm, then the wrist, and then there's the lower arm, and then there's the elbow, upper arm, shoulder, and so on.

Maybe we separate ourselves into different parts because Mom or Dad said, "Where's your little nose? Where are your little ears?" Naturally we need to learn these distinctions for communication in the world, but as we get older we seldom remember the whole picture. Our attention got hung up on the divisions. It's not that we shouldn't study a nose or the ears and their many great functions, but the olfactory sense will not work if there is no awareness flowing to it from the nerves in the cranium; the nose will not work if the mouth is always used for breathing. The interconnections are as vital to proper functioning as are the parts themselves.

As was discussed in the previous chapter, we spend our lives in two basic environments: the external one, with its changes of temperature, physical and emotional pressures, and so on; and the internal environment, which is closely associated with the inner rhythms of the organs, the cranial rhythm, and the movement of the inner fluids. As the membranes of our bodies develop from the first cells dividing the embryo to the more complex membranes that separate one muscle from another we begin to recognize our inner bodies as a safe intimate environment, while outside our skin there is an ever-changing environment to which we must constantly adjust.

These environments are kept separate and functional through membrane boundaries, the skin, connective tissues, visceral membranes, joint bursa, and so on.

Membranes are made of three main components:

• Collagen — the protein contained in connective tissue and bones, which provides strength and gives substance to the structure;

• Elastin — the protein forming the basic substance of elastic tissue, which offers flexibility, resilience, and the capacity to change and recoil after an extension; and

• Fiber — the slender, threadlike cells of nerve, muscle or connective tissue which keep the integration and connection the way the small roots of a plant hold the soil together.

The membranes, which cover virtually everything in the human system, are responsible for transferring nerve impulse into functional action. Because the membranes are heavily laden with nerve fiber, and have a vibratory resonance like that of a drum, they are very much involved with carrying information or awareness back and forth between our inner and outer environments. For example; the brain sends a message to the finger to lift; the message is received in the sheath about the bone, in the tendon connected to the bone, in the sheath around the tendon, and in the muscle connected to the tendon; if the membranes are all in agreement with no particular impairments or inhibitions in place, the movement happens with some degree of ease.

But what if that finger had been in a splint for two months because it was injured? The same message to lift comes into the area, but the awareness of the finger is now unclear, partially because of disuse and partially because the membranes have been disrupted by "mechanical difficulties." Body history, such as an injury, will cause the membranes to excessively increase their support, adding extra collagen in the area. Repeated actions or experiences often are fortified in the tissues with collagen, the hardening protective agent, for added support and safety.

Imagine being a secretary, recently promoted into the big leagues. You make more money, have more responsibility, and you know that heads roll quickly here. You're typing away and the door opens behind you; it could be the boss. Maybe you get a little tense in your belly, your shoulders lift. This goes on for months and your body tissues habitually hold the tightened position "just in case" it's the boss. You are protected, but you forget about the armoring as it becomes the "new" you, prepared to survive in the office environment. The moment-to-moment response to increase safety and support has become a long-term habitual position.

Imagine being on an assembly line, turning a bolt to the right with your right hand, maybe 300 times a day for twenty years. The wisdom of the body says, "I'm going to have to anchor in here because there's so much movement from the torso outward that something has to stabilize, has to hold home base." The membranes, full of very intelligent nerve fibers, support this action by organizing around the task, literally shaping themselves around the bones; the collagen hardens around the pattern of action and establishes a dominant pathway. That task is performed efficiently because there is a life impression built into the arm and brain. Memory has been established in the flesh.

But what happens if someone working the left side of the line becomes ill and you have to take his place? Now you have to reverse your actions, go against the grain, against your membranous pattern. You can get the job done, but not too easily or efficiently. And at the end of the day, you have pain in your neck and upper back. The pain is worse the next day, and almost unbearable by the third day. Finally, you go to a therapist who works diligently on those areas. You feel better briefly, but the next morning your chest hurts. What happened? Basically, you didn't acknowledge the life impression created by constantly turning to the right. You got the left-sided job done by compensating with your neck and back, and when the strain was released from the neck by the therapist, it went into the ribs. The membranes were just doing their job.

INHIBITION

The membrane boundaries are meant to be semi-permeable to allow access back and forth between environments, to let information, energy, and fluids pass through them and yet provide adequate protection when needed. To act in the world, or to have a well-functioning body, we must have the ability to come and go freely, to go into our core and come out again, ready to function in the world with ease. If we are to keep our boundaries free, we have to reckon with the fact that almost 90% of our neurons are designed for inhibition not to do something. It's an interesting concept. No wonder I can't dance. No wonder I can't learn another language.

This dynamic of inhibition has a very specific purpose: it stabilizes or fixes a body part or segment in place. Without inhibition, when we stretch our arm to grab a can of beans off the pantry shelf, our whole body might come along with the arm and we'd fall into the pantry. Imagine trying to type on a computer keyboard if every time you moved your fingers, your whole body came along. If we're seated at the table and reach for the salt, imagine how difficult it would be if body parts other than our arm came along randomly. Since all our parts are connected, a single movement could travel throughout our system.

Certain parts need to be restrained in order for others to work. For a sail to work on a ship, the mast has to be fixed. The sail has to be anchored to the core and then the core can be involved as the ship moves. We need to engage the structure of the legs and the large muscles and begin to connect the two with the pelvis, move the sternum and the ribs and get the skeletal muscles of the ribs to move the neck of the occipital bone; we need to get all the parts communicating and get the body core to recognize that it's okay to anchor and let these limbs move all over the place.

Inhibition serves a valuable function, yet with all that inhibition in place, it is no wonder we get so easily bound by our repetitive actions. Because of the ability of the neurons to inhibit action by stabilizing the tissues, actions that we repeat over and over again can create an habitual response of the neurons and tissues. In one sense, this is extremely helpful. We don't want to relearn how to tie our shoes every day. Inhibition has helped us with the basic function of tying our shoes. This is a life impression. And yet, what would happen if we tied our shoes a slightly different way each day? Wouldn't we create more flexibility in our membranes, have more options in the way we use our bodies?

Changing the pace at which we do something can shine the light of attention on our repetitious actions. Choosing a simple habitual act and doing it a little differently such as holding the toothbrush with the other hand, buttoning a shirt from top to bottom, reaching for the door handle with the other hand can awaken new pathways for action.

Exercise

As with all the exercises in this book, please remember this is about learning, not doing. Only work within your comfort zone; nothing can be gained through over-exertion. You don't even have to be able to reach your foot or the shoe lace; just moving with attention in the various directions will awaken the brain's nervous system and make more space in the membranes. Breathe and rest, stopping between different parts of the exercise. If any section is too challenging, do less.

Making New Pathways

Put on a pair of shoes with laces. Walk around and notice your whole self: how your feet feel, how your legs move, where you feel restricted. How about your hips, low back, neck? How do your arms move as you walk?

Get in your normal position to lace the shoes and direct your attention to the right shoe and foot. Notice: did you bring the foot to you or did you bend over to the foot? Whichever way you did it, now try it the other way. What about both ways? Could you bring the foot toward you and bend toward your foot? Making new pathways in the brain and the membranes create new ideas of how to use your body and provides access to your membrane bindings.

Try all the different ways you can imagine to get in position to tie your shoes. Do it with your eyes open, then do it again with eyes closed. Do all movements gently and slowly. Don't go all the way. Just start the pathway and move back and forth, creating a new groove in the brain and in the tissues.

Now do the same exploration with grasping the laces. Come from the front of the shoe, both hands coming in from their respective sides, feet resting under the knees. Repeat this action slowly back and forth several times. Now do it with the feet crossed at the ankle. Come to the point of grasping the laces, then back away. Do this many times with each approach. Put your feet very close together, parallel, and go for it slowly. Try it with your feet as far apart as is comfortable.

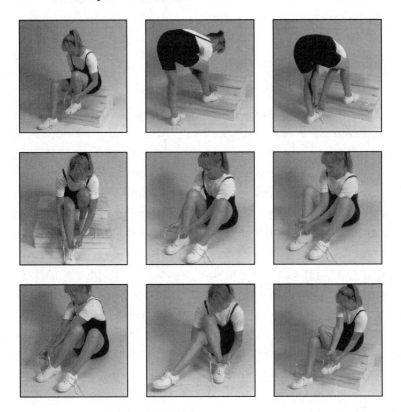

I am assuming you are in a chair. Now move to some stairs. Sit on the stairs, placing the right foot one stair lower than the left, and go through the same procedure as above. Then place the foot two steps lower and again go through the motions. Now face the stairs, placing your right foot one step, then two steps, higher than the left and repeat the procedure.

What if you did all of the above sitting on the floor? Walk around a little. Is there something different about how you move now? Compare the two sides of your body. Explore again all the areas that you noticed at the beginning of the exercise.

Follow the same procedure on the left foot.

Because of the many options you introduced into your system around the task of tying your shoes, you may now have more ease of movement in your whole self.

Inhibitions in the functions of the body, held in place by the membranes, appear also in personal behavior. We may feel like dancing but are too inhibited to follow through. This inhibition is not just shyness; it has a physical aspect. For example, the limited range of physical motion in a sedentary lifestyle can restrict the sense of personal and emotional options. A desk worker who is a practicing couch potato at home can become impeded by the "sitting" imprint. The shape that we habitually assume tends to "set up" like gelatin in a mold the membranes adapt to our habitual patterns and behavior. Living within this habitual membrane mold puts certain constraints on our movement potential. We become restricted from moving outside the boundaries of our habitual imprint.

Imagine trying to act out various feelings while wearing a wet suit that is a little too small. You try to be very exuberant but the body is held back, which tends to hold back some of the energy and feeling. If you have a desire to express joy, delight, and lightness, can you imagine how incongruent it feels not to have the freedom in your body to express what you feel within? When a small child, whose membrane package is naturally less impaired, is happy or sad, the emotion registers throughout the whole body. As life goes along, we want to be able to express ourselves in a satisfying manner. We may seek a strong stimuli a drink or drug to "loosen our inhibitions," which wouldn't be necessary if we could keep our membranes and their contents as free and unimpeded as possible so we could fully enjoy and express even the subtle delights we encounter in life.

Inhibition becomes a problem if we stay in or out too long in either environment. The membranes decide, "Well, this is what he or she would like to do, so I'll assist." Remember, the function of the membranes is safety and support.

Often the external environment serves to entertain us so well that we continue to send our energy and attention outward looking, feeling, extending ourselves and our attention for so long that we deplete the inner environment. The membranes, doing their job of supporting and protecting us, react and intensify their efforts against invasion, even from our own re-entry. Imagine coming home at night from your very high stress job. You have been so focused externally that the body membranes, being intelligent, automatically tighten a little bit, get a little thicker. The master is not at home, so the membranes lock up the mansion. When you arrive at your house, energetically, physically, and emotionally you say to yourself, "Okay, now I can rest." You lie in bed, but your eyes are wide open. Your membranes literally are not permeable to your reabsorption into inner peace. Your energy is still in the office, still talking on the phone to Paris or whatever, and you have inhibited yourself from re-entry. You can't go "home."

In a sense, the goal of this work is to be able to permeate the membranes at will, to go out and be functional in the world and then be able to return "home" without any restrictions. Problems arise when you go out and you're so busy, working for so long, separate from your inside environment for such a long period of time, that those membranes start to stiffen and thicken to such a degree that you can't go to sleep or meditate or just be at peace. On the other hand, maybe you've become so internal, so reclusive, that you develop inhibitions about moving outward into the world, about expressing yourself. Maybe you spend many years in solitude, fortifying your inner environment, and then think, "Wow. Now I'd like to go out into the world and share my knowledge." You try to interact with another person and find you're just too inhibited to share what you've learned inside.

The idea is to retain pliable, semi-permeable membranes. As we go to work in the world, we bring along something of value from our inner environment. And when we're done working, we can withdraw, bringing home some new insights for deep inner contemplation and personal growth.

We come from the West with its abundance of enchantments coming at us through the air waves, in print, in virtually every corner of our existence. One of the best ways to contend with this is by returning to our inner home, talking with God, praying, meditating, and nurturing our relationship to the inner environment. If we don't "check in" to the inner environment on a regular basis, the pathways back and forth get overgrown with nervous actions, we become estranged, inhibited, lose our inherent vitality. When our spirit connection is lost or seldom used, the well runs dry. At some point, food is not enough, exercise is not enough, herbs are not enough, acupuncture, bodywork, nothing is going to sustain us until we refill the spiritual well. We need to remind ourselves often of who we are, through direct contact with our inner source.

Can we get through our inhibition and get back to who we really are, free to choose another option in the way we live? The answer is a resounding YES. We can turn our attention away from the land of enchantment and use the uplifting vitality of the inner environment to melt the hardened membrane boundaries, to consciously set new and more flexible boundaries.

MEMBRANE HARDENING

In order to function in life, to entertain the mind, to fulfill our creative urges, and to maintain some degree of peace and connection to who we really are, we must be able to shuttle at will between our inner and outer environments. To do this, we need easy access back and forth through the membranes of the body. But at some point our membranes became less permeable because we got really good at shaping the membranes into the hardened images in our minds. How's that for getting the horse behind the carriage? If we add membrane hardening to neurological inhibition and historic imprinting, we see how we build difficulty into our systems.

Membrane constraint may be "called up" for a variety of personal needs, which all translate into a need for more support and safety. The constraints impede response and encase the awareness. The nerves get short-circuited. We get hung-up in our elements, and unawareness accumulates in the tissue bindings.

Membrane hardening begins early, back when we are learning how to use our new bodies. Lying in her crib, Jane's eyes are functional and she can turn her head just a little bit. She's having a difficult time learning to deal with this digestive stuff, but she's beginning to trust that this is an interesting place. All of a sudden there's quite a lot of noise. The vata, (the energy that relates to the nervous system air and ether), starts to become a bit of an insult to her nervous system (as vata increases, fear and anxiety may arise), then Grandma comes in with a big camera and goes FLASH!

Now, obviously, Grandma thinks the world of Jane and wouldn't dream of hurting her. But Jane has no idea who Grandma is or why she did such a thing, and her membranes around the eye, and the nerves in general, have been assaulted by this tremendous unexpected light. At this point in our development we perceive light not just visually but with our whole being. It's entirely possible that Jane's membranes tighten up a bit, her neck and eyes get that startled response so that, maybe even for a day or two, she's a little shy about anybody coming up to the side of the crib.

Years later Jane has long since lost awareness of that early event, but it's still registered in her membranes. The tissues have a very profound responsibility: if there's a strong enough perception or response to an action, the tissues start to exude more collagen the hardening agent so that the ease, the slide, the glide, the elasticity of Jane's eyeballs and facial structure, maybe even of her neck, are just a little different. She may have lost more than just pliability; she may have become stuck in the layers.

Possibly because of that one event, or maybe a number of events that continue to occur, Jane develops the idea that it's not quite safe to extend her vision or perception out too far because who knows what will happen? That concept is not registered in her intellect; the tissues have registered the belief.

Maybe Jane starts to need glasses because visually she cannot move her vision in and out with ease. Maybe she has a difficult time turning her head in one direction, or always flinches in the same direction if startled. Jane may go to a chiropractor or therapist of some sort who cracks her or pushes her tissues around in some meaningful way and she says, "Yes, that feels better." Then she signs the check and goes out into broad daylight. "Oh, bright sun," and Jane is back to where she started.

Another way in which membranes become hardened is through the body's compensation for lost parts or functions. Let's say you fell from five feet up in a tree onto your shoulder. First, you felt fear as you lost your balance, which increased air and ether, which in turn increased fear and anxiety. You hit the ground, and the tissue layers were compressed, interstitial fluids squished out from between the muscle layers, pain and more fear infused the system, particularly in the area of impact. The tissues stiffened to protect against further injury, which held the impression in the area, including the pain and the fear. Now, between the deep layers of tissue in your shoulder, lives an etched-in-flesh memory a bookmark in your living story.

When trauma is introduced into the organism, the elements are strongly effected and they increase their protective attributes. The body reacts quickly to restrict the area. If the wound is deep and the accompanying emotion is strong, a long-term recovery period is necessary both physically and emotionally. You begin to move around the area instead of using it while convalescing, initiating a chain of structural compensation. In an organic system, everything is related to everything else: any change or lost component sets a new pattern in motion or shuts down the pattern of function.

Like most habitual tissues, the injured area gets re-enforced with membrane sheathing. It's like debris collecting in a small stream which eventually grows large enough to divert the stream. The same dynamic occurs in the body. As the restriction begins to impair the functional pathway physically and then neurologically, the membrane layers become laminated and the flow of energy and/or the neurological feedback is diverted. The new path of least resistance is unfortunately less efficient than the original and will often create further compensations as the body tries to contend with the new pattern. A compensatory pattern is very different from setting up a new pattern in order to expand one's options. With a compensatory pattern there is no connectedness, just an urgent call into action. Some body part is going to have to work overtime for the immobile shoulder segment, like when a labor force is short a person, everyone else must take up the slack.

We deserve to have all of our parts at our disposal at all times. The "missing in action" areas of the body can be relocated and often brought back into the line of duty by using the body "bookmarkers", the membranes. The information that was stored in the shoulder the pain, fear, and so on can be accessed and all can be resolved when the membrane storage unit is opened and begins to function again.

Reclaiming Your Frozen Assets

Scan yourself from head to toe (this ought to be getting easier with practice). Are you holding any area of your body without reason? You may be tightening your jaw, contracting in the stomach, squinting your eyes. How about your legs and feet? Can you find any way to make yourself a little more comfortable? A pillow, better light, an arm rest? If you are as comfortable as possible with no unnecessary holding, good for you. You are among the very few. Either that, or your pattern of strain is so well-hidden that you may be unaware of it.

Have you ever been angry and found some time later that you are still holding your fists, stomach or jaw tight, or holding your breath? When you let go, what a relief! Depending on how long and how tightly you were holding, you may have felt a noticeable rush of energy when you released it. After a good session of bodywork or psychotherapy, or any therapy that helps you "let go," don't you feel more vital, more alive? You no longer have to use your energy to maintain a pattern of holding. It takes a great investment of energy to organize, hold in place, and sustain deep patterns. Think of the amount of energy contained in life impressions that have been held for years in your body, mind and beliefs.

Let's say you did some work in your attic last fall and turned on an electric heater to stay warm. After the job was finished, you forgot to turn off the heater. As the winter months passed, your finances are being exhausted by outrageous electric bills. You have forgotten that the heater is still on and using up energy. The same type of wasteful expenditure occurs when you maintain old beliefs held in the flesh.

I once had an assistant teacher in my training program, a very good psychotherapist, who, in high school, had a boy friend with the obnoxious habit of taking her by the arm and pulling her along, which got to be very uncomfortable and somewhat demeaning. As an adult, she was walking with a friend after a nice dinner, and as a friend might do, he gently took her arm. She immediately felt anger. Thankfully she had some skill in self observation; she recognized this was not related to the friend, but that she had held this well-established physical and emotional pattern in place for many years. With this recognition, she relaxed through the shoulders and chest to such a degree and experienced so much relief that she began to cry. She had been using so much energy to keep that pattern available that she was constantly feeling the drain and didn't know it. For weeks after the release of the old pattern, she felt energized.

Energy, attitudes, fluids, structural and visceral holding are all involved in the maintenance of patterns. This relates to all patterns the ones you use on a day-to-day basis as well as the ones you established when you were young, when you had that accident, when there was a death in the family, when you felt you were wronged and had no way to say it or get satisfaction. All those experiences put a claim on your energy. To hold a pattern in place for any length of time, whether it is one of belief or action, the body constructs a framework using the heavier elements. When earth and water (the elements predominant in collagen) are involved in pattern construction, the deconstruction process must be somewhat physical. Just changing your mind will not release the gathered elements.

Maybe you are in the habit of smoking cigarettes and you finally resolve, "That's it. I've had it. When I wake up tomorrow morning, I'm not going to smoke any more." Maybe you meditate on it or do an affirmation. Maybe you even go to a psychotherapist or hypnotist or a spiritual counselor and collect lots of reinforcement for "I'm not going to smoke." For the first few hours of the next day it seems you are succeeding in your resolve. You have small cravings but you overcome those with your will and your sustained energy. You decide to take a walk outside, where there is traffic going by and gas and smoke in the air from the passing vehicles. It doesn't have to be cigarette smoke, but now there is a chemistry occurring in the tissues of your lungs that has a relationship to smoke. Even your lips are responding in some way. All of a sudden the craving gets stronger and you haven't even seen anybody smoking yet. Pretty soon the craving is quite strong, and by the end of the day your resolve is fading and your body is starting to exert itself. You reach for a cigarette.

The first step in reclaiming our vitality, our "frozen assets," is to see the pattern. This requires self observation from a new perspective, as in the earlier exercises. There is a definite limit to how we can see ourselves from within our pattern; we need an objective view to change our rhythm. Shifting into neutral and accessing information and energy from the stored pattern in the flesh will help get the needed perspective.

The only way we can be free of the entangling patterns we weave into our bodies is to make a conscious decision to increase our safety and support. One way to reinforce the safety and support necessary to change a habit is to include the elements in our picture of ourselves. Think of how difficult it is to keep water in one place; water wants to flow. Ether and air are even more difficult to contain. The membrane boundaries, as well as the spaces that they define, are none other than ideas held in place by the mind utilizing the five elements of the physical plane. There are many self-liberation processes, such as meditation, Feldenkrais movement therapy, yoga, and so on. One of the best methods of awakening is through touch, because all the current information and the history is stored within the tissues.

Touch is a powerful tool because the membranes that hold habit in place are composed of earth and water, the heavier elements of the body. If you're going to liberate these heavier elements, it requires some physical contact because the membranes, the connective tissues, have hardened.

The next chapter teaches the Touch of Awakening, which

we will be using in all the treatments given in this book. Before going on to the next chapter, reconsider your constitution, think about your sensitivity. How would you like to be touched and where is the safest place? What do you feel are the reasons that you would or would not care for contact in any area? Consider the congestion of the elements, tissues, or habit patterns that may be contained. Think about the missing support that may have created the need for such a contained area. What part of your body, with what elements and what feelings, could offer enough support to let yourself go?

SECTION II

How We Change

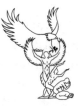

Chapter Five

The Touch of Awakening

Do not continue to live in the same old way. Make up your mind to do
something to improve your life, and then do it. Change your consciousness;
that is all that is necessary.

- Paramahansa Yogananda

SEEKING THE HEALING MEMORIES

Each experience we go through in life can be considered a
lesson. Sometimes we "get" the lesson at the time of the experience. Sometimes we store it away for future reference
because at the time we don't have enough perspective, time,
maturity, or ability to utilize the information. I like to refer to
this stored information as the healing memories.

Did you ever lose your wallet? I remember the sinking feeling as I realized the wallet held all the proof of who I was in the
world: money, credit cards, driver's license, pictures of my
family. There was the added pain of loss, making this also an
emotional injury. I searched my clothing, all the places I often
put the wallet... nothing. Then suddenly I remembered putting
the wallet in my wife's purse before she went shopping. Sure
enough, there it was. What a relief! That's a healing memory.
That pleasant sensation of security, however fleeting, comes
from the healing that memory facilitated.

We use Life Impressions work to direct us to the frozen
assets within through safe supportive touch. Once we reach

the "organic file cabinet," the membrane envelopes which contain our stored healing memories, we can use that information to update the files, the physical representations of our beliefs, feelings, and experiences that have set our patterns of behavior and self-image in place. When the files are accessed, we can throw out old outdated information, habitual responses, and retrieve the information that can lead to our healing.

Many years ago you and your partner separated and things were said on both sides that are painful to remember. Then, in a conversation with a friend from the "old days," you finally remember some of the good times you had with your ex. Other memories return and some healing takes place. This may also happen in a body therapy session when a body part is contacted in a non-invasive manner that permits the "tissue memory" held in the membranes to spring forth. Suddenly you can feel again the way someone you loved touched you in a way that made your heart open. This healing memory carries with it the joy of that moment.

I had a cousin, a bit older and wiser, who was my best friend as a child. We played together often and I began to see him in a very special light: he knew everything and could do no wrong. Then we had an argument which got out of hand and my cousin hit me on the head with a plastic gun. I was in shock. My hero, my best friend, hit me! The physical impact wasn't so terrible, but the information behind the event the betrayal of trust was. Years later, during a bodywork session that included a lot of work on my head, I reclaimed that memory. I was in tears, not because the treatment was painful, but from the stored pain of my hero's "betrayal".

The impressions from our life experiences have been folded into the flesh, along with the thoughts and feelings we had at that time. Memories which are "etched in flesh," the memories bound by the heavier elements, require touch before they are released. Ideas come into physical form in the membranes the boundaries that can harden up around ideas and habits and injuries. This is why manual therapy is so important. It's not that personal therapy or spiritual counseling can't be helpful in changing our lives, but the membranes must be softened and made more permeable in order to change on a more permanent basis.

When I first started doing bodywork, I'd dig in with my knuckles and elbows and the person would look great and feel blown away. They were opening up so fast that it was pretty exciting, but over and over again I saw that the changes didn't last. There may have been a great deal of body organization on the surface, but it was also creating a great deal of compression at the core. The more someone opens without the connection to the skeleton, the less integrity there is. I changed my approach.

In the beginning of the training for Life Impressions work, instead of using direct work utilizing, knuckles and elbows right away, I teach the indirect work, using the awareness to see what we can deal with consciously, seeking a way in to where healing can begin. After the indirect awakening, we may then use direct work as needed. For example, if we move a leg in various directions, it can release old patterns from the torso, from the spine, from the viscera. But if we don't have the awareness that the leg can move in a 360 degrees span, then moving the leg in all these directions can actually increase the strain to the body core.

We want to treat our bodies, our beings, with respect, and trust the intelligence contained within. All too often, even with the best of intentions, we become mechanical, get lost in our theories, mechanical instruments and techniques, and leave out the most important aspect of the treatment accessing the person's inner wisdom. All we have to do is access the wisdom of the body, whether through touch, herbs, drugs, needles, a kind word, or simply a gesture. We have not invaded somebody else, but are respectfully developing an environment in which change can take place. If we add respect for inner wisdom to the laws of physics, profound and amazing results can occur in terms of long-lasting changes.

TOUCH OF AWAKENING

The manner in which one is touched, the type of touch and the "response-ability" of the tissues, nerves, and brain are essential elements in establishing long-term positive change. By listening with no agenda to the recipient during the touch, we can feel the tumblers release their combination lock on the body structures that contain the healing memories stored within.

Miss M lay on my therapy table again. We had been working together for several weeks. I asked, "Are you certain you did not injure this shoulder?"

"No, not that I recall." We had been over this before. Often when you touch an area that is "loaded" or has some strong history, you can feel a certain density a clue that some event is contained in that area. As I touched the area of Miss M's right shoulder, it had that feel. I decided to stay there, just holding the area and offering support. Soon movement began from deep within the ribs under the shoulder. I followed, and more movement emerged. This continued for several minutes, then Miss M began to cry. I let this go on for a moment, not wanting to interrupt the flow, and the feelings got stronger. I noticed her eyes were closed and rapid eye movement was occurring.

"What's happening ?" I asked.

She responded from a great distance. "I remember the accident now."

I was surprised because she had never before spoken about an accident. "It was so terrible... my brother was killed, I awakened to find him leaning against my right shoulder." Indeed she had not physically injured that shoulder, but there was certainly something in there. As the session went on, many "kinks" came out of the shoulder, ribs, and spine on that side, very spontaneously and with great feeling. At the end of the session, she had cleared a major block in her body and in her life through uncovering the healing memory.

The point of this story is that when the time is right and the support and safety are adequate, the elements that store our life impressions separate and let the information come forth. The key in this case was touch the Touch of Awakening. The Touch of Awakening conveys support and offers safety. It's a touch for listening to the body versus touching to do something with intention. Often, because there are no expectations, we feel safe and have just enough extra support to take a good look inside.

If the elements in our system are in relative balance, our nervous system sends clear signals that indicate what is acceptable and safe and what should be avoided. Vata (air and ether) responds to any stimuli by moving the awareness from place to place through the system. It's like having the house alarm turned on; entrance is gained only when the right code is entered. "Is it safe? Do I have enough support to receive this?" If someone touches you, instantly the nervous system determines the quality, intensity, attitude, and safety factors relative to that touch. If by chance the touch hits a sensitive place on your body, no matter what the intent or attitude behind the touch, you will recoil.

Miss M, for very good reasons, had blocked out the accident. As the years passed, the tissues and elements of the body coalesced around that stored event and packaged it so well that it was almost inaccessible. Touch of Awakening offered the right conditions for opening to a healing memory. Built into the Touch of Awakening is respect, safety, and support. The respect is based on the fact that whatever is contained in the body, however it has been shaped and built up the elements, there is a good reason behind it somewhere in that person's history.

Touch of Awakening indicates the type of touch we want to use in Life Impressions work: to stimulate the process of self-correction within another individual without making a big noise outside; to bring forth inner knowledge pertinent to one's well-being, growth, or healing through manual contact; and to facilitate the release of information, fluids, and functional capacities for self-healing. Otherwise, we're just pushing tush, so to speak. If we're going to work on somebody else, it's important not to have an agenda of what we think they need. If we have too much of an agenda, we're not going to permit the wisdom within their bodies, within their minds and spirits, to emerge. There is a balance to be struck in reading the "living book": 50% listening/50% intervention.

Some years back, doctors who were affiliated with the New England Journal of Medicine did an experiment on warts, using every mild non-invasive therapy possible. They finally resorted to meditation and hypnosis, suggesting "Your wart is gone." Many people did lose their warts. Being a medical organization, the scientists tried systematically to determine: "How did the mind tell the body what to do? How did this happen?" The people whose warts went away were from all walks of life. Most had just a basic education, yet every one of them had the intelligence built into their systems to get rid of the warts. The intellectual and highly educated scientists couldn't figure out how to explain what had happened.

In Life Impressions work, we treat bodies as if they were intelligent. They are profoundly so. That's why the Touch of Awakening can work. The nervous system responds to touch; proprio-receptors talk to the brain and give back stories about what occurs. A body is so incredibly intelligent that just approaching its vicinity produces a response: "I like, or don't like, this person." "He's coming at me too quickly, or too slowly." "She's very tenuous." All this goes on before we even touch the body. Imagine what happens when a therapist approaches a body and is thinking: "Ah, this is a pitta guy. These guys are always stiff in the joints and I'm going to just rub it this way and that way." Without the therapist saying anything, the client's body already senses that the therapist has an agenda.

Maybe he had absolutely the best intentions. Let's say a cervical vertebrae is leaning in the wrong direction and he knows this vertebrae needs to be moved back. But the client's body, in its own intelligence, in its own wisdom, is saying: "Well, yeah, but before it goes there it needs to come back here further and go around this way and then go forward and then go back and then I can use it." Or, "This vertebrae could be more useful over here, but I can't have it here because my pelvis is over there and it doesn't have any support." There are no useful changes possible without adequate support and safety. And even with adequate support and safety, if change is imposed, even though it's well intended, it may not be used because the client didn't learn anything. The recipient must experience and participate in the change on some level.

We're going to develop our Touch of Awakening in a very specific fashion so that how we touch liberates great potential for well-being. Until there is enough safety and support, until the nervous system and brain know that there are new systems in place that are better than the old ones, until the kinesthetic sense feels the connection throughout and all systems are GO, there will be no lasting change. Some may say, "Oh, that's some kind of cosmic or spiritual idea or airy-fairy stuff of the New Age." This is not what I'm talking about. Touch of Awakening takes into consideration the bio-mechanical components that make up the system, the elements that compose it, the energies that run through it, and beliefs that are essential to sustaining it.

You may not be a manual therapist, or have any interest in becoming one, but because you have a body and loved-ones who you want to support in the best way possible, you may want to know about the Touch of Awakening. All the preceding information in this book was designed to prepare you for the idea of touching non-invasively, with a deep respect and a degree of understanding as to how we got the way we are, what keeps us that way, and finally, what we need to change. Consider for a moment your new understanding of how a life impression is made, the development of boundaries, the way in which the elements are in concert with the needs of the person, the environments and their influence on us: all these ideas are inherent, nothing new. We are reminded of who we are. In essence, if we trust ourselves, we can get better. What could be easier?

We are connected from head to toe, core to surface, back to front, and inside out by the membranes. The membranes are full of awareness because of the nerves imbedded in them. The entire human organism is permeated with the five elements, two of which air and ether are very subtle and permeate all aspects of being. The elements of air and ether are responsible for the sense of touch and govern the nervous system. With all these factors in place, touch becomes a profound awakening tool.

Touch can get our attention. Think about tapping someone on the shoulder to get their attention. You have a specific purpose, and may tap with a certain urgency, or vitality. On the other hand, if you are looking for a spontaneous response from them, one that may lead to healing, the tap-on-the-shoulder type of touch would be inappropriate. We want a touch that can get through to them and yet have a neutral charge. If we want the touch to enhance well-being, it must carry those special qualities of non-invasiveness, safety and support.

Whether you are experienced with touch in a therapeutic manner or not, begin with a fresh mind, as if you have never touched a person before (I recommend this to all my students, and practice it often). If you begin with a clean slate, with no agenda and great curiosity, you will be more receptive. In some ways, if you have very little experience, you have some advantage with this type of work. For those with past bodywork experience, once you get out of your own way and the client begins to give you information, your "data base" of techniques will be very valuable.

When we touch another person, we can't be saying to ourselves, "I want to do something nice for this person. I know just how to fix this," or "I don't know what I'm doing and since I'm such a klutz I can't possibly do anything right." It is not up to us to do anything, particularly with this type of touch. We're just touching to get their attention. Physiological, structural, bio-mechanical, and elemental results will transpire, based on the interactions of the brain, nervous system, the relationship to safety and support with any type of contact.

Have you ever watched a water bug skimming along the surface of the water? They're pretty big bugs, but they don't sink. They contact the water so gently they ride upon its viscosity. That's how we want to initiate contact in the Touch of

Awakening; we want to ride the surface, the viscosity of the flesh. We want to feel the resonating response to our contact, like landing on the surface of the river of life. We are composed of approximately 70% fluids (blood, urine, lymph, etc.) channeled into rivers of life by the membranes, with spaces for the rivers of prana or energy. With that in mind, we're going to imagine that the flesh we slowly contact is the surface of a river and we're going to sit there ever so lightly. The recipients awareness becomes, "Aah, what's that I feel? Oh, it's okay, my viscous shield is intact. But since I've been alerted, let me go about checking myself and self-correcting."

Consider the make-up of the person you want to touch. If their tissues are dense, as with the kapha person, you may need to contact them more strongly. If the vata person is fearful and anxious, you may need to touch very lightly. If the person is irritated, agitated, or in an analytical state, such as a pitta person, you may have to contact them slowly but firmly. However, people don't always respond in character, particularly when in difficulty. When the normal responses to problems don't work, i.e. the characteristic response, we try other ways. Therefore, when contacting someone, it is important to always start in neutral, gently resting on the surface of the skin, and wait for a response.

Begin with an attitude of non-doing, curiosity, and caring. Be willing to be guided, to listen and follow the recipients body as it expresses its needs. Imagine you are a safecracker and there are many alarms in the layers of tissue you are about to touch. There are, after a fashion, alarms based in the nerve-laden layers and in the historic imprinting. As with any combination lock, there is a precise sequence that must be activated to release the "goods." If you sensitize your hands and listen very carefully, you can feel the stages of release calling.

There is an added advantage to this "living combination lock." If the recipient feels an initial sense of safety, you can make some mistakes and the system will be very forgiving, continuing to make self-corrections very gracefully. Remember, you are working with awareness, not just tissue layers, elements, and energy.

Exercise:

The Touch of Awakening Sequence

Make contact: Lay your hand on the person's forearm. (I choose this place because it has many noticeable layers, is generally distal to the more complex structures, and can offer an avenue of release for the larger parts of the body.)

Contact as a water bug would land on the water, very softly, so as not to break the viscosity of the surface. At the first touch of your hand, vata (which governs the electrical and nervous systems) responds the air and ether elements take notice, the electrical currents of the body are interrupted, and there is an instantaneous evaluation based on the nature of your intent and the response of the relationship between the inner and outer environments, of which you are a part. Decisions are made regarding acceptability of the contact. If you are offering the "Touch of Awakening," the response very likely will be neutral or somewhat pleasant and safe, permitting a continuation of their evaluation and self-correction process.

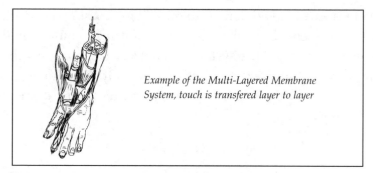

Example of the Multi-Layered Membrane System, touch is transfered layer to layer

Listen: Listen with your hand and heart. This is a "felt" sense of listening. Your non-invasive, supportive presence will have an effect based on the brain and organic response:

• At the neurological level, recipients will perceive the added support and safety and very likely relax a little, (the first tumbler in the lock begins to yield). There is a learning that begins in their system about relating to themselves in response to an increase in support. The system may well go into search mode, investigating where it might find more within itself.

• At the elemental level, the added support and the heat from your hand will have some chemical action on the tissues. The kapha or collagen may begin to become more gelatinous, still retaining its ability to support but not restrict. The temperature is registered just under the skin. This may begin to respond to both the heat or cold contained within and the heat from your hand, causing a new balance in the local temperature, thereby affecting the pitta balance. As the pitta (fire) responds, a chemical change is forthcoming. This is a self-regulating action, self-correcting if necessary. Meanwhile, you are doing nothing, or so it seems.

• At the structural level, all layers, including the bone, have their responses to the more superficial response and the personal feeling response of the recipient. The

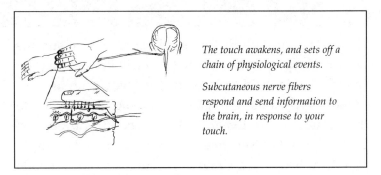

The touch awakens, and sets off a chain of physiological events.

Subcutaneous nerve fibers respond and send information to the brain, in response to your touch.

layer of fluid under the tissue that is most directly under your hand becomes more responsive and moves better. This movement is discernible by you.

Follow: In some ways, you are just along for the ride. Follow the flow set up by the bio-mechanical actions of the consciousness and elemental transition. If you cannot perceive the subtle actions under your hand, (this awareness can be developed with practice), instigate some very subtle directional inquiries. Note the term "inquiry." We are not making demands on the system, we are asking for directions. Slide the surface tissues; they are more free to glide because of the melt down. Gently move your hand side to side or up and down. This action must be just slightly perceptible to the person under your hand, otherwise he or she may feel coerced and set off the alarms. Determine the direction of ease and slide the tissues in that direction ever so slightly. Wait there for further instructions from the person's body.

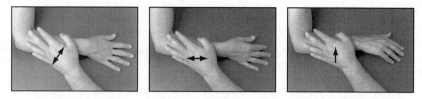

Sink, settle in: With the bio-mechanical actions and the personal responses to contact, there will be some significant change in the density of the local tissues under your hand. This permits your hand to sink slightly deeper into the tissues of the forearm. At this point you are just under the pitta layer; fire is held just under the skin to maintain body temperature. There may be a subtle change in the person's overall temperature, sometimes a slight flushing, some heat being discharged, a sense of coolness, or no awareness at all of this action. In some very sensitive people, the whole system may respond. As you sink, be very respectful; you are being invited into the recipients temple. Have a sense of reverence, and don't go in farther than you are invited. When you hit the next layer, stop at its surface and rest there in neutral.

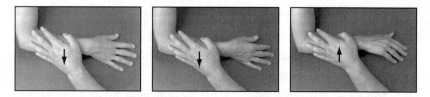

Call and response: At this point hold your position and call for movement from the recipient, a very slight action similar to your own entrance into the system. (This is an opportunity for the people receiving the work to treat themselves gently and with reverence.) Initiate movement from the bone by having the person rotate an arm to bring one of the bones upward and the layer of tissue under your hand. Active participation establishes awareness and functional potential in the region, the self-image is enhanced, and the recipient actively takes up residence in the limb. Very slowly, have the recipient return to "neutral." Repeat this several times, then have the person rotate the forearm in the other direction.

Return to neutral: Slowly rise out of the system, permitting the tissues to "fill in" behind your hand as it moves toward the surface of the body. A dry stick that has been held in a deep pool of water will not rise directly, but will wobble slightly on its ascent. In this same way, your hand must lift out of the tissues, noting and following the drifts of fluids on the way out. The more clearly and exactly you emulate their pattern, the better will be the outcome of this mini-treatment.

Remove your hand from the body: You are still in the field of the recipients body even after you are no longer in physical contact. The energy field, vata , flows through and around the form.

Explore the difference: The person receiving the work can now move the limb about very slowly and subtly, along with the other one that has not been worked, and note any differences.

The brain and nervous system learn by comparing differences. Based on how these differences feel, how easy they are to use and maintain, and the safety and support factor, this new way of acting will be explored by the recipient and may be implemented in other areas as well. Why would you move with effort on one side when you have learned how to move with ease on the other?

However, just learning how to do something does not mean that it will automatically happen in other places. If a life impression has been solidified in the form, you must re-establish the functional ability, sometimes by melting down the elements with stronger contact, sometimes by processing the feelings, beliefs and thoughts behind the pattern. Complex fixations, ones that involve loss of function, elemental congestion, belief system impact, and so on require addressing the human system in different ways to satisfy the need for change and to release the healing memories.

There are many variations to the Touch of Awakening which we will explore later in the book. Practice the Touch of Awakening for some time so that you become comfortable with it. It would be advantageous for the TOA to become second nature, but not automatic. You always need to be present and automation leaves the human element out of the equation. You want this to be an act that can stop any tendency toward mechanical application.

THE THREE TYPES OF TOUCH

The Touch of Awakening can be further refined. There are three types of touch according to Ayurvedic medicine: Tamasic, Rajasic, and Sattvic. Although they are three different specific types of touch, for our purposes consider them as variations on the Touch of Awakening.

The tamasic touch is a strong, solid contact which is offered to break up congestion. It is a touch that is said to go beyond the mind, or one might say beyond the mind/body established barriers. It then lets the mind "catch up" or re-establish a new boundary, one that is more fitting to who you are now. It is my feeling that although it may be a strong touch, it need not be painful. Pain reduces the willingness to learn and re-experience the "positive" changes they may reveal. One can be touched deeply with gentle non-invasiveness, and there is such a thing as "good" pain, or letting the pain out, or changing one's relationship to what is thought of as pain to intensity.

Tamasic relates to the ultimate contraction, the necessary boundaries that are thought to be needed for life in the physical world. As we find more support in life from aspects other than the gross form, we can afford to upgrade the contractile quality of the form. Tamasic can also be a concept, or generally a force in the universe. One can behave, eat, think, or speak tamasically. For example, speaking tamasically is effective in getting someone's attention (although the response may also be strong). The pitta person often uses this manner of speech. Depending on the person spoken to, this manner of verbal contact may elicit a strong response anger, fear, or resentment.

Tamasic is a manner of contact or action that can break the ice, penetrate the density, or melt the congestion, but must be used appropriately. The tamasic touch is often used with the kapha constitution, or on areas in the other constitutions that have developed a non-responsive, static, congestive, and basically kapha-genic quality.

The second type of touch is rajasic: a touch of movement. It is offered at a pace that permits the mind to stay with the contact, testing and yielding its own boundaries. It can initiate integration, flow, blending. The rajasic touch can release the ultimate in expansiveness. There is a time for contraction and a time for expansion; knowing when to use the various types of contact is a job of listening. The rajasic touch stays in tune with the person; it does not push the envelope. The safety that it provides may encourage the recipient to expand limits and break contractile boundaries. The rajasic touch generally

increases heat, which can melt the old beliefs and body patterning. Often when there is a trauma of some nature, the body
membranes will isolate or encapsulate the area, thus creating
separation (a tamasic state) an interference in the flow of movement, energy, thought, or feelings. The best type of touch for
this pattern may be rajasic, applied in a gentle awakening manner.

Quite often, one may be inclined to use more than one type
of touch. For example, when the area of encapsulation is well-
established, a tamasic touch may be used to "break the seal,"
then a rajasic touch to expand and integrate. This combination
may be helpful for the pitta person if applied well. You must be
careful not to fan the fire, as when there is too much congestion
between head and heart or when the heat is drying and contracting the body.

The rajasic touch can also be applied to vata people. They
can examine their boundaries and even pull them in, but the
offering touch must be done very slowly. Remember the intelligence in the tissues and the fiber. Like the child's toy the
Chinese handcuff that when stretched will then recoil further
this is how one may use the expansive rajasic touch with the
naturally expansive vata person. In general there are clearly
times when each touch is of benefit for each constitution.

It is most important to begin contact in such a way that you
permit response from or "draw forth" from the recipient the
right type of touch. This is best done using the principles of
Touch of Awakening, which will call for more specific touch as
your skill at listening increases. Recall the basics: increasing
safety and support, building trust and a willingness to make
change. Then the organism will divulge its need and you can
offer the right type of touch.

The third type of touch is the sattvic: a very subtle touch, sometimes referred to as the spiritual touch, or touch of balance. By polarity, tamasic has a negative type of electrical response or contractive, and rajasic has a positive type of electrical charge which is expansive. Sattvic is the neutral charge. A touch to bring subtle balance, the sattvic touch can work with the para-sympathetic and the sympathetic systems. This touch can bring balance to the pulses. If tamasic is contractive and rajasic is expansive, sattvic is oscillating in balance.

Because of the gentleness of this type of touch, it may be applicable when other types are unacceptable, and certainly should be mixed into most treatments as the need shows itself. In general, this touch is the best for the vata constitution. As we all are at least part vata, and vata is resposible for 60% of all imbalances, it is good for most people.

The following exercise demonstrates experientially the differences in the three types of touch.

Exercise

The Corn Starch Exercise

Very slowly, mix two boxes of corn starch with warm water, a little at a time. Add more until you get a consistency like thick pancake batter. As it is in the body, the consistency is very important; too much water and the responsibility will be reduced, too little and the consistency will be too dense.

After the mixture is right, let it set for a few minutes. Now try a tamasic (or what we might refer to as direct) contact. Press your fingers into the mixture with some force. Try to reach the bottom of the bowl. Vary your pressure and the speed with which you press. The faster you go or the more pressure you use, the more resistance the corn starch will provide. This is just the way our tissues respond to invasion too quick, too hard, and they resist. Ease back out about halfway, then pull hard trying to get out quickly. Again, your movement will be impaired relative to the pace you use. In the human body, it is just as important for you to ease off on the contact as it is when you make the contact.

Try the rajasic touch. Gently contact the surface of the corn starch. After making contact, begin to wiggle your hand as you penetrate, noting how much easier you can get to the bottom of the bowl. You are enhancing the expansion potential of the material. The human body is much more responsive than corn starch. Consider the inner relationship or "dialogue" you can develop working with the system versus on it. Use these types of touch to create a language for communication.

Now just lay your hand on the surface of the corn starch. Your sattvic touch should begin to sink your hand effortlessly into the mix. This is the same as making contact, the first part of the Touch Of Awakening. With the corn starch, the heat and weight of your hand are enough to cause the response and the settling in. In a living body, the awareness, coupled with heat and the increase in support and safety, cause the collagen to melt.

For a more interesting exploration, try making a mix that is dryer (more vata) or wetter (more kapha). You might let the corn starch sit for several hours and separate, as elements might separate in certain conditions like edema in the ankles. With a gentle manual mixing, see what it takes to get the consistency to return.

Another practical example is to drop some small item into the corn starch mixture and go for a search and rescue. The point of the exercise is not to disrupt the corn starch, but to pluck the item out as cleanly as you can. As you withdraw the item, explore the rajasic wiggling to get it to come out clean.

Mrs. J came in to my office in North Hollywood some years ago, having been referred by a psychotherapist. She stated that she was very sensitive and that she could barely stand to be touched, but felt the need to have some work on her body. She felt she was "losing touch" with herself. Was there anything I could do? This happened before I knew about constitution, elements, or the three types of touch, but I always knew how to listen.

I asked about her history. She answered, "I was molested as a child and it continued for many years." I considered this a very good reason not to want to be touched.

I asked about any other significant history. She withdrew slightly, tightening her shoulders and collapsing into her abdomen. As I observed this I said, "It's okay if you don't feel like speaking about it now." I had found early in my practice that safety and support were the main tools for any positive change.

To my surprise she relaxed, length returned to her torso, and her breathing got fuller. I waited for her to make the next move. Finally she said, "The abuse was ritualistic and sexual, a cult, very evil." A chill went through my body; I had to breathe a few times to clear my own stuff. She continued, relating some other details of her history, and then slowly got more current.

"About six years ago I had a total hysterectomy, and two years ago I developed breast cancer in both breasts and had a double mastectomy." I began to realize how touch could be very inappropriate, and was learning more from her then just her history. What pain and shame she must have endured, and the manner in which she was trying to get it out of her body by literally having the experience cut out.

She had finished talking. We both sat there a few moments in silence. Finally, when it seemed appropriate, I asked, "Now that all that history has been awakened, how do you feel about working with your body?"

"I'm scared."

"That seems reasonable to me," I said. "Is there something I can do to make you more comfortable?"

To my surprise, just that statement caused her to relax. She said, "I'm not used to doctors (although she knew I was not a doctor) waiting to hear what I feel before doing something to me."

I simply said, "It's your body and your treatment session. I feel I must hear from you about what we are to do." This seemed to amaze her to no end.

"Well," she said finally, "I feel better already. When do we start?"

"We already have," I said. "Shall we explore touch?"

"You have me curious about it although I am a little frightened." She lay on the table.

I said, "Where would be the best place to start?" Again an amazed look and a pause.

"My feet."

"Tell me how it feels as we make contact at your feet." As I came closer to touching her feet, I could feel her pull away, so

I stayed just 1/8th of an inch away and said, "How about if you touch me with your feet?"

A pause, then she began to reach downward and contacted my hands with her feet. A very slight sigh escaped her throat.

"Are you all right?"

She began to cry softly and soon said, "It feels good." The session went on in that way having her create the touch, and on occasion exploring what it was like for her to be touched.

I offer this story not to show what a great therapist I am. Quite the contrary, I had no idea what to do. In fact I simply got curious, listened, followed, and then had her create her own therapy. In a sense, I followed all the basic things that are included in the Touch of Awakening.

Interestingly enough, we explored to her delight all three types of touch. At times she would push very hard or ask me to press harder; at other times we barely connected tactually. This was my first introduction into the principles of the work I now share in classes and in this book.

PRACTICAL APPLICATIONS

As we delve deeper into the theory and practice of this work, do not lose sight of the goal: to touch not only the flesh, but the spirit within the tissues. Therein resides the source of our well-being. This is the point of the practical work. There are techniques by the hundreds, but technique alone will not foster healing and awakening.

When someone needs a helping hand: hold one hand on the area of the heart, the other on the back directly opposite it. Make appropriate contact, wait for a breath or two, then settle in and follow any subtle movement you perceive. At the end of the excursion of movement, hold your place there for several breaths and listen for any other movement, a sigh, any "signal" regarding change. Return to neutral. Note any change, follow with a hug.

When there has been an injury and it is appropriate to make contact, contact the person ever so softly. Listen. How can the area be supported? What is happening under your hands? Is it expanding, contracting, hot? Remain in the same position, hands gently surrounding the injured area, just offering your presence. An area of trauma will always have a vata energetic disturbance. Soft containment which increases the local security can sedate the area and help stabilize emotional response. After several minutes, move one hand to a place above and the other to a place below the area of injury and again make contact. From these two areas, sink and follow movements. Exaggerate the movements very slightly, hold, return to neutral. Check in with the person and repeat as needed.

During times of emotional stress, the breath and the mind are first to be disrupted. The best way to settle the mind and emotional body is through the breath. Once again, vata will be disturbed (60% of all imbalance is due to vata because it controls the mind and nervous system). Ask the person to lie down. Make non-invasive contact with both hands on the chest. Wait for several breaths, then gently follow the breath with your hands. This will slowly draw attention to the breathing and, in many cases, ground the person or at least provide support. Soon the person will feel safer. As safety and support increase and are noticed, the emotional pattern will subside, not because you did anything but because they were able to return to "home base." If further work is necessary, go to the abdomen and repeat procedure.

For a digestive disorder: place all five fingertips (the fingers represent the five elements and can stimulate subtle currents) around the navel, as close to its center as possible. Make contact, listen, sink. Wait a breath or two between each phase of the treatment. Follow the "drift." There will often be a subtle glide in some direction; slowly track it until it stops, (no more that 1/8th of an inch). Wait there (you may begin to hear gurgling noises) for three breaths, then return to neutral. Repeat this process one or two more times following other "directed movements."

If any problem is serious or persists, see a qualified medical examiner.

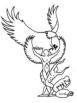

Chapter Six

The Components of the Human System

After many years in the field of bodywork and personal development, I came to the conclusion that most methods of working with people were of some value. The determining factor was which method or system best fit the needs of the person in question. To determine this, I would always evaluate the person based on what type of structure he or she had, the density of the patterns, and the person's ability to receive the work. It wasn't until I studied Ayurvedic medicine that I found better tools for reading the "living book". I soon found that if I put together all the observational, palpatory, characterological, and constitutional factors, and listened to what the person had to say or to what was being said behind the words, that "reading" became easier.

We already have the Touch of Awakening, with its listening and following, as a basic treatment tool. In order to get a clearer understanding of the way in which the Touch of Awakening can help to update our life impressions, it is necessary to be able to picture the components that make up the human organism and how they relate to each other. What is the body composed of, and how do the components work? We may be somewhat aware of the basic functional elements from the Western viewpoint of anatomy, and may even have some idea of how the nerves, muscles, bones, tendons, ligaments, organs, and so on work. But to give us a fresh perspective to work from, let's look at the development of these components from the Ayurvedic system.

In the Ayurvedic system, all life is composed of the tridosha, the triple conjunction of vata, pitta, and kapha working together to build and maintain the human form. From the very subtle aspects of vital energy to the more gross manifestations and actions that we exhibit in life, the tridosha are in concert at all times.

AYURVEDIC COMPONENTS

To understand the components of the human system from the Ayurvedic perspective, we must look again at how the tridosha vata (air and ether), pitta (fire), and kapha (water and earth) combine to create the various tissues that in turn shape the person. The following brief explanation of the subtle essences of vata, pitta, and kapha covers only a small part of the very complex and profound system of Ayurveda. All these aspects and functional actions of the elements are combined to make larger more complex structures, the tissues. For a deeper understanding, please consult more complete Ayurvedic texts (see Resources).

I studied the five elements for several years in acupuncture school. The Chinese system was difficult for me and I eventually dropped out of the training. I must be a Hindu at heart. When Dr. Lad started to talk about the elements in his Ayurvedic class, I thought to myself, oh no, here we go again. Then Dr. Lad began to chant (much of the traditional teaching is from short verses in Sanskrit that tell the story of the medicine). I began to feel the elements, not think about them. Sanskrit is a profound and beautiful language that is based on vibration more than on the intellect. Just hearing a Sanskrit chant can be uplifting because of the manner in which the sound of the words affects our inner being. The following Sanskrit names are difficult to translate and may have no equivalents. Enjoy them.

The Five Subtle Forms of Vata

Vata divides itself into five aspects, or directional flows, each with its own special action and direction.

(1) Prana is centered in the brain and moves downward toward the lungs and heart. It governs all higher sensory functions: sight, hearing, taste, touch and smell. Prana also governs swallowing, inspiration, the intellect, and consciousness. In short, prana brings the energy necessary for those vital functions down into the body.

(2) Vyana is centered in the heart and governs all circular motions: the circulation of blood and lymph, the circular motions of the joints, and the circulation of prana itself. Vyana works along with prana to create the functions of the heart. If we want to make a circle with our arm, vyana must be present and functional in our body to enable the circle to occur. Without the downward aspect of prana, vyana will not work.

(3) Udana is situated at the region of the diaphragm and moves upward. It governs the expiration of breath, coughing, speech, vomiting, jumping, hopping, hiccuping, and all upward movements, including the movement of the soul out of the body at the time of death. Udana is helpful with memory, as it returns energy to the brain.

(4) Samana is situated in the abdominal region in the small intestine and enables linear movements, such as the side-to-side action of the small intestine. Samana also controls secretions into the stomach, the peristaltic action in the intestines, and other side-to-side movements.

(5) Apana is located in the large intestine and moves downward from there into the legs. It governs all the lower downward actions, such as defecation, urination, flatulence, expulsion of sexual fluids and the fetus; in short, all the functions of the lower pelvic cavity and into the legs.

The Five Subtle Forms of Pitta

(1) Pachaka is the fire of digestion. It is located in the stomach and small intestine. In the West, we would say we need certain amounts of hydrochloric acid and other digestive juices for proper digestion. This is true, but before that we must have the subtle energy of pachaka, otherwise we have a collection of juices with no power to interact. The five subtle forms of pitta are vital essences and qualities; they are less a tangible substance than a force in our inner life.

(2) Sadhaka is the light of intelligence, located in the brain and heart. In the West, we consider intelligence to be located in the brain and don't often confer with the heart when establishing beliefs. This type of pitta determines truth or reality as it deals with mental digestion.

(3) Bhrajaka, located under the skin, governs the temperature of our bodies and maintains the luster, complexion and color of the skin. Flushing, blushing, or paleness can relate to the increase and decrease of this pitta essence. Movement and food in the system may keep us warm, but we would still be cold without the force of bhrajaka pitta under the skin to "ignite" the body heat.

(4) Alochaka, located in the eyes, is the fire that is responsible for receiving and processing light from the outside environment. Once again, it is the power to process the light not the light itself.

(5) Ranjaka is the fire that makes color possible. It resides

primarily in the liver and spleen, although it travels about in the blood and bile. You might even imagine the shape of the liver like that of a painter's pallet .

The Five Subtle Forms of Kapha

The elements that compose kapha are in themselves more gross than that of both vata and pitta. From the Ayurvedic perspective, we now are getting more solid matter relative to the components of the system.

(1) Tarpaka is the white matter of the brain, the nutrition for the nerve cells, the nourishment for all the sense organs and the cerebrospinal fluid (the carrier and sustenance for the intelligence). It stabilizes feelings and provides emotional calmness.

(2) Bodhaka, located in the mouth, enables the taste through the saliva, softens the food for digestion and adds subtle digestive material.

(3) Avalambaka, located about the heart in the pericardium and in the lungs and pleural membranes, is responsible for lubrication of the lungs and heart. It is the main kapha of the body, giving energy to all the other kaphas.

(4) Slesaka, located in the joint spaces, is the lubrication (synovial fluid) for all the joints and gives strength to the joints.

(5) Kledaka, located in the stomach, protects the lining of the stomach from the strong digestive juices and liquefies food for continued movement along the digestive path.

All well-being begins with attitude. Like any organism we only work as well as our subtlest parts. If the tiny bearings that help start up a huge machine are out of order, the machine won't run. In the human body, according to Ayurvedic medicine, order in the system begins at the level of thought and then moves into the energetic levels. Once the vital energies are in motion and moving in the right directions cooking our food, igniting at the right time, nourishing and lubricating they carry information and nourishment, establish easy and efficient patterns of function, and provide the building components for the layers of tissue that we work with in our daily lives.

The system next develops into seven layers of tissue (the dhatus) which build, nourish and sustain the body. Each layer provides sustenance for the next layer and is, in turn, supported by the layer underneath it. For example, a healthy, well-developed lymphatic tissue nourishes the next layer, that of the blood, and the blood, when healthy, keeps the lymph system strong. It's like gardening. The compost matures and is placed on the garden to eventually nourish the plants, a layer above the composted soil. In their cycle, the plants die and become more compost. If the compost is too hot, it may burn the plants. If the blood becomes too hot or toxic, the lymph system will have to work much harder and may itself fall prey to disorder.

It is said that it takes five days of healthy eating, thinking, and lifestyle to produce the essential substance for each layer, and another five days for that layer to help build the next layer, and so on. Thus in thirty-five days, with all conditions being met, all seven layers may be rebuilt, from the sexual tissues, the deepest layer, to the lymph system, the most superficial layer. Because all layers are interconnected, any positive response at any layer of the system will reverberate to all the layers in the system.

As we look at the developing complexity of the human form, let's remember that all structures, from a single cell to the entire skin covering the body, are contained in membranes which are connected to one another and the brain through a network of nerves and consciousness. That which we are, the spirit behind the material, elemental, and mechanical workings is not this collection of parts.

As you read about the seven tissue layers, consider your own history, especially in reference to the given symptoms and treatments. Do you remember having such symptoms and wondering what to do? If it should happen again, you can think differently about your situation and find a quicker solution. Think about which layers in your body are overdeveloped or underdeveloped. Can you see why you may have had problems with respect to that pattern? For example, if you develop too much muscle (mamsa), you may have problems in the joints when the fat lubrication layer is squeezed out. Certain tissues offer a more natural ability to be soft or forgiving. See how this is applicable to your body or that of another.

My suggestions for hands-on work, for coaxing the life-force to awaken, are measures which assist the individual to self-heal. This therapy is not designed merely to alleviate symptoms, but to treat the whole person. The following information allows us to build a data bank for understanding the symptoms an individual may divulge during the listening phase of the work. To me, the greatest error in the healing arts is to develop a static treatment system. One cannot treat by the book, but purely from the personal level.

The Seven Tissue Layers

(1) Rasa is the first and most superficial tissue layer. In the West, this would be the lymphatic system. Rasa begins to set up the order in the garden of the body, nurturing the other tissues and being nurtured in return. The main location of the lymph system is around the heart. Since lymph is one of the substances in the body that must be circulated, its location is the same as vyana, the vital air in charge of circulation. Rasa,

or lymph, is circulated throughout the entire organism. It is a viscous, white, oily substance that contains some food essence. Psychologically, rasa promotes calmness, quietness, softness and happiness.

Symptoms and Treatments: An excess of rasa would produce nausea, excess salivation, heaviness in the heart, edema, coughing, coldness and shortness of breath. This might indicate the need for tamasic touch to break up the congestion and some rajasic to expand and increase the heat. A deficiency of rasa might produce weakness, dehydration, heart palpitations, and a sense of emptiness. Treatment would include sattvic touch to draw in and balance. Other treatments would include herbs and dietary considerations after a careful study of pulse and other characteristics. This is true for all seven tissue layers and imbalance descriptions.

(2) Rakta, the blood tissue, is the next building block of the human system. Rakta contains a little more earth and fire energy than rasa. Rakta tends to be hot, red, light, mobile, slightly oily, and sticky. The main location of rakta is in the liver and spleen. Psychologically, healthy rakta enables warm feelings, freshness, ambition, an ability to expel anger, brightness, and delicacy. Healthy rakta can be established in ten days.

Symptoms and Treatments: Excessive rakta produces a fullness in the veins, redness in the eyes, rashes, itchiness, gout, dermatitis, and headaches. The sattvic touch can be used to soothe the fire. A deficiency in rakta might produce roughness of the skin, cravings for acidic foods, slack blood vessels, shortness of breath, and palpitations. A rajasic touch would be expansive and heating.

(3) Mamsa, or muscle tissue, is the next layer. It is composed mainly of earth and water. Some of the qualities of mamsa are slow but strong movements, bulkiness, softness, and oiliness.

This is one of the layers that gives shape and strength to the body, offers protection, and has the ability to do work. In the West, we find mamsa or muscular tissue attractive. Mamsa is mainly located under the skin and with the ligaments. Healthy mamsa tissues psychologically produce forgiveness, bravery, strength, and straightforwardness. It takes fifteen days to produce healthy mamsa tissue. Mamsa protects and nourishes the next layer, that of the adipose tissues.

Symptoms and Treatments: Increased mamsa can produce full buttocks, lips, pelvis and arms, general heaviness in the body, and muscle tumors. The tamasic touch can help restore some depth to the layers and better hydrate them; the rajasic touch can expand and increase vitality. Having too little mamsa tissue leaves one weak and vulnerable, often having to compensate by increasing nervous energy or mental development for sustenance in the world. A diet of foods that can build more muscle, and exercise to create strength can be of help (see Bibliography, *The Ayurvedic Cookbook*). The type of touch one might find valuable will depend on what type of compensation has taken place. In general, the compensation would require sedating vata, thus a sattvic touch would be of value.

(4) Meda, the adipose (fat) layer, is composed mainly of water and earth. The characteristics are: heaviness, oiliness, slow semi-liquidity, and softness. Meda lubricates all tissues, keeping bones soft and pliable, and giving strength to the bone tissues. Meda also adds lubricant to the eyes, nails, teeth, and stool. Its main locations are in the suprarenal glands and kidney area. Healthy meda can be created in twenty days.

Despite the great stigma in the West caused by the fat layer, it is absolutely necessary in the functioning of the human organism. The relationship of how much fat one should have for health can vary greatly. We have long been "fed" images by the fashion industry, the entertainment industry, commercial television, and the diet industry as to how we should be shaped. It is no wonder the pitta type became the ideal body. However, for many of us this means neglecting our natural constitution. Note carefully the following characteristics and balance them against the need to be svelte; perhaps you may develop an appreciation for the "fuller" form. The psychological characteristics of healthy meda are love, compassion, delicacy, and abundance.

Symptoms and Treatment: Excess meda can produce a fullness in the flanks, buttocks, and breast; oily skin; breathlessness; profuse sweating; and lung congestion. A tamasic touch is helpful to reduce congestion and break up stagnation. Rajasic touch can reduce density, enhance expansion, and increase metabolic activity. Deficient meda produces emaciation, emptiness in the joints, pain in the pelvic bones, and a craving for kapha.

(5) Asthi, the bone tissue, is composed of the elements of earth and air. Its general characteristics are dryness, solidity, roughness, heaviness and a static state. The asthi tissues provide support to the whole system and give the body a functional shape. This layer nourishes the next layer, the nerves. Asthi tissues create hair, nails, teeth, big sturdy joints. The main seat of asthi is in the pelvic girdle, the sacrum and ileum. If we have a good quality of asthi in our system, psychologically we have a supportive nature, leadership qualities, are hard workers, helpful, and have an ability to be forgiving. The individual with strong asthi will be tall and straight, with big nails, large teeth, and thick hair. It requires twenty-five days to produce healthy asthi tissue.

Symptoms and Treatments: Excessive asthi may produce excessive ossification in the bone, extra teeth, abnormal bone development. Tamasic touch breaks up ossification and congestion in the joints; sattvic work balances the information in the system. Deficient bone tissues may produce aching pain in the bones and joints, weak teeth and gums, general dryness, weak nails, loss of hair, and brittleness of the bones. Rajasic work with warm oil can expand and lubricate; sattvic work will sedate the vata.

(6) Majja, the bone marrow, is related to the nervous system. Composed of water and air elements, the majja maintains the qualities of softness, oiliness, liquidity, slipperiness, and delicacy. It offers support by filling the spaces in the bones and softens the joint spaces. It originates in mammary secretions and offers nourishment to the sexual tissues. The main location of majja is in the bones and joints. The psychological characteristics are: happiness, strength, compassion and caring. It requires thirty days to produce healthy majja tissue.

Symptoms and Treatments: Increased majja can produce heaviness in the eyes, enlargement of the small joints. A deficiency can produce osteoporosis, spontaneous fractures of the bones, and pain in the bones.

(7) Shukra, the reproductive tissue, is composed of earth, water, and air. Its physical qualities are: liquidity, oiliness, sliminess, and mobility. It will not generally form until around the age of sixteen in the male, when it forms white ojas (protoplasmic matter). In the female body, maturity is reached at thirteen years and shukra forms red ojas. The main location of shukra is in the testicles and the ovaries, and all over the body. Strength in the shukra dhatu enhances the psychological traits of happiness, joy, compassion, inner beauty, vitality and intelligence.

It takes thirty-five days to form healthy shukra tissue. Note the amount of time necessary to replenish healthy reproductive tissues. Expelling the sexual fluids to excess is like pulling the plug on all the other tissues in the body. There will have to be compensation on some level of the tissues when the deepest layer is being drained. This is one reason that yogic lifestyles encourage sexual moderation or celibacy. By the time all seven layers of tissues have produced this high quality substance, it contains all the elements of vitality and life-force.

Symptoms and Treatments: Excess shukra in the male produces an excessive flow of semen and the formation of stones; in the female, it produces excessive menstrual flow, tubal pregnancies, or miscarriages. Deficient shukra may produce pain in the penis or scrotum, incapacity for intercourse, scanty semen or blood, dryness in the mouth, and general malaise.

A WORKING MODEL OF THE BODY

Whether we build with elements and attributes, as the Ayurvedic system does, or cells, electrical impulses, and biochemical actions as we do in the West, the outcome is eventually the bones, muscles, membrane layers, and so on, the components of the body, which become the pages or book markers in the "living book." In order to have a working model of the human body for making corrections in the system during treatment, we use these components and their relationship to the inner and outer environments so we can adjust, reposition, or bring them into our awareness, making life in the body more pleasant. Add to this the possible modifications in behavior, emotions, and general qualities of each person and you can begin to "read" yourself and others more fluently, keeping our life impressions malleable so we are free to learn and grow.

As we develop a working model for further consideration and treatment, keep in mind that we are directing our attention to an organism in space that has to deal with gravity and many other forces, an organism that must be able to move freely and still have adequate stability. We are not just this organic framework of living components but a living, breathing person, with fears, beliefs, misgivings, constitutional predisposition, habits, and old life impressions congealed in the flesh. The mission, should you accept it, is to find the optimum support from your organic system and healthy beliefs and ground it all in an awareness of who you really are.

The following is a quick review of the components of the system, combining Eastern and Western perspectives.

We are composed of:

Consciousness: which comprises all. In this model, it is the variable that can be called upon to make changes in the "hard copy" by increasing awareness.

The Five Elements: the first step down from consciousness into the world of matter, from the subtlest energy particles to the bulk of our flesh, we are these elements.

If we want to change any pattern we must tend to consciousness and the elements. The rest of the components are different from both the traditional Western view of structure and the Eastern view. Please bear with this development. The multi-layered organism of the human body is vast and complex. The following model helps us to locate where we are in the system of our living human book.

The linear part of our minds needs something to hang its hat on, and we also need to be able to locate where we are in the system and what "part" needs to be supported. In essence, we make the parts clearer so that they may evolve into the whole more gracefully. Any part that does not work well hinders the organic whole we seek. In truth, after consciousness and the five elements, we are an organism whole and spontaneous, with no real borders. But be kind to the manner in which we were educated. The "cylinder model" provides a functional idea of how the human system might be differentiated, and how we might interact with the differentiated components to make life better.

If we dissect the body, we will find bones that seem to group together to form sections or cylinders.

The Three Cylinders: the first cylinder is composed of the sacrum, spine and cranium, and is somewhat separate in its encasing membranes.

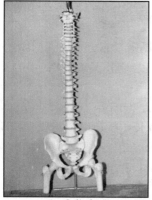

1st Cylinders

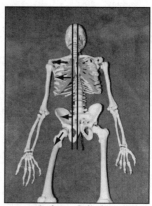

2nd two Cylinders

The next two cylinders, parallel to the main cylinder of the spine, cranium, and sacrum, are each composed of one-half of the shoulder girdle, one-half the rib cage, one-half the pelvis, and one lower and upper limb. (see photos above)

The Outriggers

Can't find that name in your anatomy book, can you? Picture yourself in the South Seas. You're going to haul your goods to the next island in a hollowed-out canoe, but the seas are high and hitting you from the side, and your canoe always tips over. Your wisest tribesperson notices that while swimming, if she holds her arms in against her body, she goes straight down, but if she holds her arms out, she has more buoyancy. The same is true while floating. If she floats with legs and arms open, she can ride the waves. The tribe, being open-minded and seeing a better idea, puts pontoons, or outriggers, on the sides of the canoe. Outriggers are like the long pole given to a tightrope walker to provide more lateral stability. And sure enough, the outriggers take the waves and leave the canoe more stable. What makes this work so well is the fact that the outriggers widen the base, increasing support, and are more flexible than the central canoe, leaving the center of the canoe more at ease. Exactly what we want in our body!

Looking at our anatomy more closely, starting with the foot and hand, we can see that there may be a similar arrangement in our structure to the outrigger on a canoe.

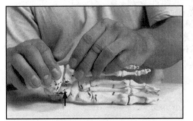 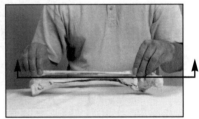

Foot Outrigger   *Lower Leg Outrigger (Fibula)*

If we follow up the leg or arm, we see that the bones of the lower part of the arm and leg are divided, providing outrigger space, that wider base of support, and adding a more flexible lateral aspect of the limb.

Generally, we want stability in the center and more mobility on the outside, with the capacity to shift when needed. What if we really want to flex the spine and it has gotten all that stability frozen into it? We need to be reversible. But in general, if the outer portion of the foot is very pliable and mobile, just like the pontoon on the boat, if it can stay really elongated, then when the waves hit, the people and cargo in the boat of our body stay dry and safe.

The Ball-and-Sockets

The ball-and-socket joints are another major aspect in the components of the structure. Think of the torso as a flexible rectangle with the ball-and-socket joints as the corners. As strains are applied through the limbs, these "corners" mobilize to disperse the weight through the body along various lines of force. If the strain is too much, the ball-and-socket compress into the torso rectangle, and squish the other structures contained within. Think of these as reference points along the torso rectangle and their degree of mobility as a reflection of the balance between the torso and limbs.

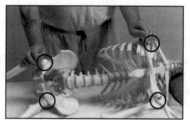

Ball & Sockets Components

The Girdles

The shoulder and pelvic girdles connect the cylinders across the midline and act as stabilizers for the weight-bearing tasks we undertake. The shoulder girdle might be thought of as a yoke, like that used by a milkmaid to support her buckets of milk. The yoke was a structure that extended the distance outward from the shoulders to aid in carrying buckets. In a sense, we have our own yoke built onto our thoracic cage. The pelvic girdle, when working well, becomes the center of power, transmitting strength from the legs and pelvis to do the heavy work in the world. Often both girdles get buried in the tissues

The Girdles

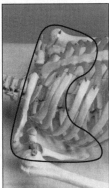

between the spine and the extremities and are lost to us, both in our self-image and in function, eventually causing injury.

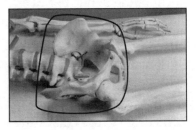

The Membranes

In general, the membranes, permeated with nerve fibers, surround all inner and outer structures; in fact, the whole body is contained in the membrane of the skin layer. The membranes are like spacers for the components, pagemarkers in the "living book" (see Chapter Four).

The Inner Membranes

There are "inner" membranes which are very complex and have many functions; they are referred to as transverse restrictions or diaphragms in some systems of treatment. (Please refer to other texts for more specific information on visceral manipulation and craniosacral therapy.) In general, these membranes lace the longitudinal structures together and provide support for various inner structures. Like most membranes, they act as functional fluid pumps in the body. Along with the other membranous layers in the human system, these inner membranes must be semi-permeable, strong yet flexible, and neurologically accessible for the components that they encapsulate. All the components of the system must be adequately spaced apart, or differentiated, so that they may do their job.

The pelvic inner membrane or diaphragm gives support to the pelvic organs and the structures that pass through it, such as the rectum, psoas muscle, and others. The pelvic membrane anchors the pelvic bones and lower spine from within.

The respiratory inner membrane supports the lungs, pericardium, and heart. It also stabilizes the structures that pass through it, such as the esophagus and various veins and arteries.

The thoracic inlet, the dome of the lungs, extends across the top of the shoulders, supporting the torso and neck and all the vertical structures that travel to and from it.

The cranial membranes, including the floor of the mouth (the soft palate), the roof of the mouth (hard palate), and the complex system of the cranial vault membranes.

The Basis for a Balanced System

Let's look at our system from a logical linear perspective, first considering the membranes. There must be adequate space in the enveloping container for any component to function well, and the quality of membrane must be supportive, accessible and sustainable. If we can begin with healthy membranes, add flexible outriggers, and the ball-and-sockets stay mobile (not transmitting too much strain onto the girdles), in turn, the girdles are able to work to their full potential, leaving the cylinders free to function with ease. This means that in treatment we can start from the inside out, making room in the system through hands-on work or movement therapy, or from the outside in, clearing the way for the inside to emerge. Where we start has to do with how people are organized, their constitution, and what they perceive as safe.

We have established many patterns in our bodies and minds, many of which have become hardened in the tissues. We get along with these impairments, but at what cost? What are the structural ramifications of imbalance? If you are forced to carry something very heavy on your right shoulder eight hours a day for many days, your natural organization will weaken because the right shoulder ball-and-socket can no longer resist the burden and will begin to compress into the shoulder girdle. As we lose touch with any of our components for whatever reason, an intricate dance of compensation takes place. The girdle, in turn, begins to yield and gives in to the right cylinder, which in turn begins to "lean" on the spine, causing it to sidebend. Now you have a scoliosis of the spine and the backaches which go along with it. You may seek treatment for the spine, but even if the spine is adjusted, how about the "domino effect" of the other components, and the membranes that contain and sustain it all?

There are any number of scenarios that could be constructed using the components other than the model I have proposed. Although understanding the interplay of our constituents can be interesting, it all too often removes our attention from the source of the pattern:'us' the ones with the fear, the ones in search of support, the prodigal children looking for the way back home. Don't forget that the components themselves are none other than our own energy, beliefs, and elements in a more solid form. If we give these structures too much validation, we get stuck and think that this is who we are something solid, unchangeable, fixed. For example, if you feel you must contain your feelings for fear of the consequences, you will need to wrap some of your inner membranes around the feeling to contain it. If it's a "gut" feeling, the respiratory diaphragm and the pelvic membranes may be called upon to encapsulate the impression. As they are drawn into this new tack, they must pull inward, distorting their hold on the rib cage and pelvic bones and possibly drawing them inward in an impairing movement. This gives the ileum and lower ribs less inside-out potential for expansion. The girdles and ball-and-socket components must compensate, and a new pattern of function, or should we say dysfunction, emerges.

As we continue to look at how we can reclaim our healing memories from storage in the components of our system and in all aspects of our life, as we learn to be more free in our movement between the environments, we have to maintain a balance between the spontaneous and mechanical aspects of life. It may be true that we can just change our beliefs and free ourselves to some degree from our own dilemma, but once the heavy elements have hardened, they must be dealt with physically. Life in the world is played by the rules of the physical universe.

Imagine looking at a person who must carry a large weight on his right shoulder at work: from the back, the right shoulder will compress against the rib cage, which will soon start to impose itself on the spine at a diagonal toward the left hip. The person is very likely to develop a left hip problem, not as a result of the left hip, but because of the hip's association with the weight bearing down on it from the right shoulder. Imagine how rotations in the system, caused by holding one hip higher or one shoulder lower, can influence the human body. How unfortunate it is to go to a bodyworker because you have a pain in the spine and have only the spine worked on. Not that the spine doesn't need to have some attention, but the spine is in core relationship to many layers that reside on top of it. If you treat the spine and don't deal with compensations in the cylinders and in the membranes, you may even do the person a further disservice.

We've got to look at a lot of levels all at the same time, listening with our hands. If we use the Touch of Awakening, all the layers are dealt with simultaneously. It doesn't relieve the bodyworker of the responsibility to understand the mechanics of what he or she is doing, but it gives more potential for helping with a very simple approach. If we just add support and safety to a system, then problems have a chance to self-correct. If we add safety and support and a Touch of Awakening, we're really giving clients a lot to work with.

For those of you who are anatomists, let's take a short trip into the orthopedic model of function for a moment. The basic support for many, many components begins with the outriggers. If you have an adequate differentiation between the lateral and medial arch of the foot, this results in adequate functional movement in the fibula, calcaneus, and navicular (for those not familiar with these terms, let's just say some of the outrigger parts), and more mobility in the greater trochanter where the outrigger meets the outer cylinder at the hip. If you don't have that arch span or outrigger extended, your pelvic structure and low back will often take up the slack.

Another way to think about this is imagining a tight rope walker who has lost his pole and must grip for all he is worth to the midline, creating more strain in the middle of his body. When outrigger structure is properly mobile, it keeps the hip from sinking too deep into the pelvis and locking up the ileum so it can't move well. In turn, if the outriggers do not work, the hip begins to bury itself too deep into the ileum, the ileum gets locked up on the sacrum. If the outriggers do not work, the hip may begin to bury itself too deep into the joint of the ileum, to increase stability, the ileum may then get locked up on the sacrum, then the sacrum often moves in place of the trochanter, because it's ability to move has been lost in the joint compression. If the sacrum is locked up and forced to move excessively, every time the tightrope walker takes a step the fifth lumbar rotates laterally excessively, which it is not designed to do. Sounds like trouble! And there are a great many hip replacement surgeries every year to prove how much trouble. I'm not saying we can avoid all hip surgery. I'm just interested in helping people avoid such things if possible by taking better care of the components. As we continue with the treatments and movement explorations in the following chapters, you will have more choices as you learn that these parts of you exist.

As you can see, when we get into the orthopedic view, things gets really complicated. We don't have to know this information if we understand the concept of width and mobility on the lateral aspect of the body. The following exploration is meant to help find and improve the functional capability of the outriggers, which provide the width and mobility to support the body. The best results come from the inner awakening to the possibilities, not so much from the actual doing. So make it easy: prop yourself up with pillows, do less when necessary, or if it is too difficult, just imagine it. If you can imagine it, you are already forming the blueprint for the action. The vital airs are set in motion, which in turn set the stage for the heavier elements to glide into action.

"If you can not imagine doing something, you cannot do it."
Moshe Feldenkrais

Exercise:

Outrigger Exercise

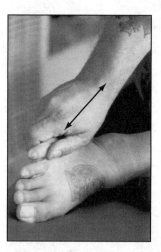 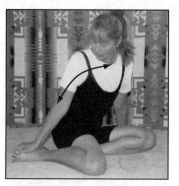

Take your socks off and sit sidesaddle, with knees pointing to the left. Grasp the outside edge of the little toe and metatarsal. Your arm is just a connecting link; this is not a stretching exercise. If you roll forward, then the foot rolls forward. If you roll backward, the foot rolls back. Lean to the left and back while maintaining your hold, the toe and metatarsal spread slightly away from the next toe.

If you're leaning so far that your foot is coming off the ground, you're doing way too much. Play with small movements. The feet are very neglected. Go to the little toe and just fiddle with it. What you're doing is including more of the foot in your self-image, extending the outrigger. Keep moving side to side.

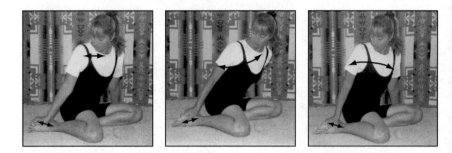

Slide your hand back so you're contacting the side of the foot just under the ankle joint. You are now holding the metatarsal bone of the small toe. Work your way backward to the heel, then stop moving. Lie on your back and rest. Notice any differences.

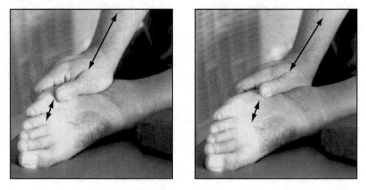

[As you lift one component away from another, it separates and creates space between those two components, which immediately gets filled with fluid and consciousness. So the changes you're making are not just neurological. They're also functional, mechanical, structural and elemental.]

Sit up in the same position and grasp the "ring" toe. Begin to lean to the left and slightly forward, then to the right and slightly backward. Do this several times, noticing how your ribs and spine participate in the movement. Slide the hand back toward the foot so you are holding the metatarsal (you are in the seam of the outrigger). Continue rocking and move your hand back to the ankle. Stop, lie on your back, rest and note differences.

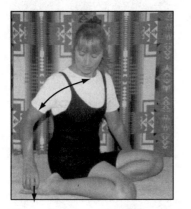 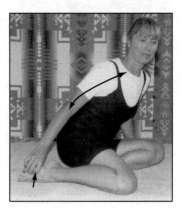

Sit up and assume the same position. Grasp the second toe and the little toe at the same time. Explore different movements with your torso, keeping the hand connected. Stay relaxed and savor the movement. Rest when you need to, then work your way up the metatarsal. Lie on your back and note differences.

[Assuming you are doing this without strain, this movement can help with knee problems. You are restoring the lateral mobility of the foot and, as an added bonus, the hip side opposite is being mobilized. Both of these actions reduce the strain on the knee.]

Come back to the same position. Grasp the right ankle bone with your right hand. Begin to lean forward and back, taking the bone with you (the lateral malleolus). Note this is a very short exertion of movement at the bone. Remain in contact with the bone and change your torso movement to a circle. Do the same movements at the other end of that bone near the lateral side of the knee. Rest on your back, then get up and walk about, noting differences.

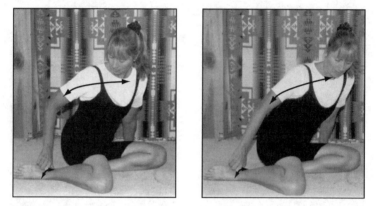

Do the other side. Explore variations in movement, such as reversing the circle, etc.

If you were gentle and followed your own inner directives about taking care of yourself, you should feel pretty good in that right foot and leg. If you can have someone else read the instructions to you or make an audio tape, you will be better able to relax. Or you may send to the Institute for cassettes and/or videotapes of all the exercises.

If possible, get a partner to explore the second foot. Whichever foot you just worked on, lie on that side. Bend your knees. Make yourself comfortable by using a pillow under the head and maybe one between the legs.

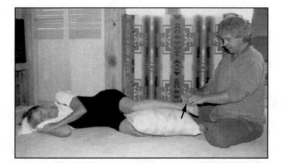

Practitioner, grasp gently and lift the lateral metatarsal and toe away from the rest of the foot, then take it in various directions, forward and back, etc. This is done very gently; you should not be lifting the foot off the pillow, just making space between the two metatarsals and toes. Now do the same movements with the second toe and metatarsal. Rest.

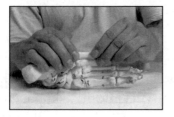 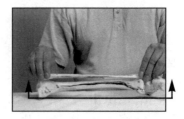

In the same position, move on to grasp the two ends of the fibula. Gently lift the bone off the side of the leg, then mobilize very slowly, doing short spans of movement in various directions. Don't forget upward and downward toward the head and foot. Recipient, take a walk and notice the differences.

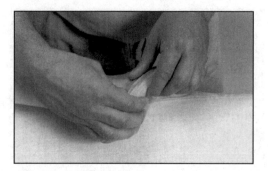

The outriggers have begun to expand. This action will tend to "run" up the side of your body to the other structural aspects of the outrigger. You now have a better base for the whole organism.

Note: I can't overemphasize how important it is to be gentle. When we're working at this layer, this is work in a body, not on a body. Working in a body requires respect and care; it requires that you work very small and slow.

By enhancing our outrigger stability and width, by having more of a foundation, even just a sixteenth of an inch more, our core components viscera, spine, sacrum, and cranium, etc., like the cargo in the boat are safer. In general, the components relate to one another in the following way: First of all, there must be adequate membrane space and support all through the system; second, there must be communication between all parts; next, the structures most external from the core need to be most mobile, and progressively moving inward there needs to be more stability. All of this requires reversibility. Remember our consciousness, because we are that, and take the time to focus yourself in such exercises and mini-treatments; many of the details of correction are set off spontaneously by our own inner wisdom.

Now that we have established some points of reference the components of the human system and gained new perspectives on understanding ourselves, we can begin to address our outdated life impressions. We can actually intervene with our established patterns and enjoy the changes. As we embark on more techniques, don't forget our main purpose, to return to who we really are. It's not about a specific technique, for techniques are a dime a dozen; it's about safety, support, and awareness leading us back to our true self.

Chapter Seven

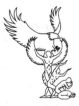

Intervention

*Medicine may chemically help the blood and tissues, use of electrical
devices may also be beneficial. But neither medicine nor electricity
can cure disease; they can only stimulate or coax the life energy back
to the neglected diseased body part. The introduction of a foreign
element, be it medicine or electricity or any other intermediary aid, is
undesirable if we can manage to use the life-force directly.*

- Paramahansa Yogananda,
Scientific Healing Affirmations

Generally, the bio-mechanical and chemical activity in our
bodies happens smoothly, unless there is an overload in the tissues. It doesn't matter what created the overload; too many
actions taking place or too many layers of information. When
there is no more room in the local area to process that much
data, or there are too many conflicting tasks taking place, the
information gets pushed into the tissues and the local area
becomes frozen. It's like hitting too many keys at once on an
old typewriter; they all lock together. Now the deeper layers of
tissue become overburdened. If enough information is forced
into the tissues, who we are is overwhelmed by what our bodies must do to deal with our current problems. We get confused
by our day-to-day experiences and lose our center, forget who
we really are and become one with the drama.

This means it is time to clean house, to update the files
stored in the body. We ordinarily see ourselves from the per-

spective of our usual self-image; many needed changes go unnoticed, and undercurrents of discomfort and discontent remain. This is where a fresh look can be of assistance a technique of observation that offers a new perspective, one with built-in constraints that demands that we reach out, move, or view ourselves differently or the assistance may take the form of another person who may help us make the appropriate changes through proper intervention.

In this chapter we look at how to build a treatment procedure based on the needs of the individual, how to awaken and enhance the life-force of those with whom we work, as well as our own. We look at the structure of the human system, searching for the "missing dimension," that part of the awareness that may be held separate from the whole, tied up in the life impressions of a time long since gone by.

We are residents in these bodily houses, living within the bone and muscle structure, the elements, the thoughts. We are not the concise, solid material we often believe is reality. In Ayurvedic medicine we are taught that all flows from spirit into matter and back again. Spirit is our source, the main ingredient in the healing process. Although we refer to the components and intervene with the pattern of their organization, remember to appreciate our greatness in spirit.

THE SPIRAL AND THE VECTOR

While I was working with a client, we began to speak about computer communication networks. As the work and our conversation continued, it became clear that what we were trying to accomplish with his body was to get all parts "on-line," communicating with one another so that each part was included in the functioning of the system and no one part had to work excessively. In order to get our whole self on-line, functioning at optimum capacity, we need differing approaches to any given situation. It's like opening a combination lock. If we want to open the lock, we use the precise actions and digits to get the proper end result. Being a mechanical item, the lock responds as planned, assuming we get the correct order. But if we apply what works in the mechanical world to the organic human system, we may not get the same results.

There are two main pathways we can use when doing bodywork: the vector and the spiral. A vector is a calculated direction, or plan of action, designed to get us to the goal most directly. The spiral is an indirect approach that is often more efficient and requires less energy. Think of walking up a mountain. The most direct route may be straight up the side of the mountain, but we will have to expend a great amount of energy and rest many times along the way. If we use the switchback trails on the mountain, a more spiral pathway, it is easier and more acceptable to our bodies. Essentially, both direct and indirect approaches to bodywork should be considered, using a blend to find the least effortful pathway, which is what we want to accomplish when intervening with an established pattern in the human system.

Let's say we have a client with a twist in the neck, the 7th cervical vertebra is rotated to the left. If we use the direct vector approach, we may go about addressing the errant bone, applying the corrective measure in a very straightforward manner. Sure enough, the bone is now in the right place, but is it congruent to the whole system? By changing one part, troubled as it may have been, have we increased the ability of the whole system to integrate or have we simply created more disturbance? Maybe the direct move on the vertebra was the very best action we could have taken, or maybe we needed a more indirect approach to gain the attention of the whole system, building safety through awareness as well as structurally.

Mr. C came from Philadelphia to see me for a knee and shoulder problem. He said, "My body therapist said that my shoulders were slumping forward because of weakness in the rhomboid muscles." He continued, "Based on that information [a direct or vector type analysis], I decided to strengthen that area on my own. One day as I worked out, I lost control of the apparatus I was using to strengthen the rhomboids and injured myself."

As I examined Mr. C, I found that the "weakness" was coming from the membrane surrounding the shoulder, which was laminated to the ribs in the back and could not lengthen. In reality, the area was not weak, but impaired in its function. A muscle's ability to be strong has to do with its ability to lengthen and contract; if either aspect of that dynamic is constrained, the muscle will test weak. With all due respect to the therapist, the tissues could not do their job and thus would show up as weak or, more accurately, ineffective.

The more attention we pay to a single part of the structure, the more likely we are to miss the big picture. By widening the search, taking the scenic route, the switchbacks, we can appreciate the whole pattern, get curious, listen, and follow the system. Why is it doing what it is doing? Instead of assuming that something is wrong, granted the part or area might not be working efficiently and might even be causing pain first, we need to appreciate that there is a need for the muscle to do what it is doing. By thinking in this way, we not only respect the wisdom of the present organization, but we can begin to get the proper sequence of treatment intervention. We may indeed need to deal with the rhomboid muscle, but only after dealing with the constraint on the whole shoulder girdle.

When we develop an appreciation of the current organization, we can reach an understanding about making positive changes to this structural arrangement with adequate safety and support. The key is to use both the vector and the spiral approaches. It's how we get to the correction that makes all the difference in a person's ability to accept long-term change, and, more importantly, to learn from the correction. The spiral method is the "smell the roses" approach; we both learn and enjoy the transition. The direct, mechanical approach leaves the recipient still ignorant of how they got that way, and thus stuck with coming to a therapist to fix it again and again.

Mr. C unfortunately had been left with the idea that one part was wrong and could be made right by strengthening. As I worked with Mr. C, I watched the way he moved his shoulders. He didn't include much movement in the rib cage. I saw that the solution to the problem was not in the rhomboid, but in the use of the rhomboid and all its associated structures. By helping Mr. C include movement in the rib cage along with the actions of the shoulder, soon the overworked rhomboid found the support it needed and graciously yielded to the assistance. It was important to note the symptom, but the resolution to the pattern came from the non-linear spiral flow around the point of fixation.

Our world of matter follows the laws of physics. But in treatment we must include the person, which most often means going at the problem in a spiral, roundabout manner that respects the fact that we have a relationship with the problem. Even if we have a straightforward impact with no emotional implications, once it's in the body, we develop a relationship, which now makes the problem somewhat spiral in nature.

We must let the clients know that they are a part of the correction. The psychological community calls this humanistic psychology. In essence, intervention needs to be a 50/50 relationship between the vector idea of mechanical specificity and the spiral development of the new relationship that will emerge from intervention of any kind. If we get too mechanical, too deep in the vector mentality in our treatment, we leave out the most essential element the person who learns nothing and is even inclined to re-create the same situation to get the missing lesson. On the other hand, if we spiral too much, spend too much time "smelling the roses," the treatment and the client are ungrounded.

In this book we refer to human experiences based on lost, stored, or misunderstood intelligence/information, and show how we may reclaim this inner wisdom or assist others in doing so. Therefore, most of the treatment work in this book is designed to be indirect spiral in nature, catalytic to the individual's self-correction potential. In general, this is safest method to apply. It offers the least offense to an organized system and avoids any dogmatic assumptions on the part of the practitioner. Using spiral or indirect treatment has a generally positive effect on the entire system, particularly the nervous system the intelligence of how we organize. But if that intelligence is overcome with effort or congestion and is not on-line, we may need to break up the pattern using very direct vector-style technique.

Let's say that the wheel of a car is showing signs of dysfunction. We can consider the inner workings of the wheel the bearings, the core structures, the inner subtle mechanisms in the machinery and this would be like dealing with the indirect or inner system, the subtle things most directly under the control of the nervous system. If we get that right, many of the superficial symptoms may disappear. Fix the bearing and the wheel rolls smoothly; release the impaired core skeleton and the gait is smoother. Get the energy or life-force flowing, release the belief system, clear the emotional block, and the inner workings of the person in turn free the outer.

There are certain cases where the spiral, or indirect, method of treatment will be ineffective and may even create more confusion. If, for example, we find that the car's fender is bent in on the wheel, no amount of bearing adjustment will deal adequately with the problem. We must get the fender off the wheel first, then attend to the finer levels. Do the direct work first, break up the congestion, unbend the dented fender so the wheel can join the rest of the system.

Direct work often employs the tamasic touch and uses the vector-type strategy to make room for order to emerge. Indirect work most often employs the rajasic and sattvic touch, and is applied with the spiral strategy. Vata is responsible for 60% of all maladies in the human being, primarily because of its relationship to the mind, emotions, and nervous system. When vata is running unchecked, most of our work needs to be indirect in order to sedate and gain control over the vata in the system. Vata also creates problems when it is contained and unable to circulate, in which case we apply direct or tamasic work. If we can maintain our vata, we have a much better chance for joy, clarity, and peace in our life, as well as ease of function in the body.

With the spiral approach, the nerves unravel patterns in the tissues and the energy which is thus released must run its course. Kinetic energy, or fire energy, is set in motion and needs to fulfill its intended purpose. Fire always wants to expand, and this energy will seek release. If it cannot be released because of a strong impairment (emotional and/or physical), then the energy may become encapsulated and become a problem. With this in mind, we need to know that too much subtle indirect work does set kinetic energy in motion, which needs to move.

The work offered in this book, although mainly indirect, is designed to work in a precise manner in accordance with the seven component layers of the system. If you practice as instructed and do not overdo it, there should be no problem with excessive kinetic energy. Direct work requires closer supervision and training and is not within the scope of this book. Specific training in all the appropriate methods is available (see Resources).

HEALING BY FEEL

To help people heal themselves, we need to go back to self-image. One of the best ways, I think, is kinesthetic, because touch is a powerful learning tool, dealing directly with the imprinted material in the "hard copy" of our body. The body is incredibly honest. It either works for you or it doesn't. The body is composed of the heavier elements of earth and water, and is subject to the laws of the physical world. You must work within those physical laws to make changes, to infuse more consciousness, to make a less dense form. To do that you must first get the attention of the body through touch.

When I was working in a Jungian therapy clinic in Denver, a psychologist referred a client to me, an elderly woman who had a problem with her left eye. For ten years she had had to tape her bulging eye shut so she could sleep. She had tried every possible therapy to relieve the problem. I had been in practice long enough to realize that some things are very difficult to correct and failures are possible. I figured if every other therapy had had no positive effect, why would my work be of any value? With some trepidation on my part, we began a series of treatments. After the second session I began to work on the head in various places, using the connective tissue work I had learned at the Postural Integration training. This was before I had any training in cranial work with the Upledger Institute, or any idea about the Touch of Awakening. I just knew I had to listen to her, not just to her words but to her very structure, if I was to learn what should be done to help this person. I didn't know what else to do. You might say my mind was in neutral with no agenda. I just began to listen with my hands and to follow as directed, coupled with my knowledge of anatomy relative to what the system was revealing.

I felt I should work very gently, therefore I barely touched her head; the last thing I needed was for her eye to pop out completely. This idea of working gently came from my understanding that a system under pressure (the eye bulging out) is quite vulnerable structurally, and from an inner sense of her delicate state. As I rested my hands on her face, I began to feel movement under my hands. At first I thought I was imagining the movement, but there it was again, like something melting, then gliding. I followed until the movement stopped, then moved my hands to another place, based on my understanding of the structural relationships of the human head. This went on for half an hour. When there was no more movement, I stopped and said the session was done. I was slightly embarrassed to take her money; after all, I had hardly done anything. In fact, I thought she might call and complain.

The next week she came back looking quite different, her eye had receded back into the socket. Obviously thrilled with the outcome, she broke into tears, and talked on and on about how I was a miracle worker. When she finally settled down, I could honestly say I hadn't done anything. This was my first experience with this kind of work the listening and following spiral work with a direct clear vector order. In essence, I had stumbled upon a new method of treatment, combining the direct use of the laws of structure and the indirect response of her organism and all the wisdom it contained.

When you develop a data bank of knowledge about the components and laws of the human system mechanical, structural, elemental, and energetic then stash that information on the back burner, allowing it to be called forth by the needs of the client. If we stay out of the way of the healing process and yet follow the rules of the physical plane, order in the system returns; it's natural, not miraculous. Know why you do what you do, based on the wisdom coming from within the individual and the laws of the organic human form. As the previous story indicates, don't try to do too much and don't underestimate the wisdom residing in all human beings.

Touch is a vata response that is very mobile and relates to the brain and nervous system. With the brain, nervous system, and the more dense body all on-line, the possibilities for improvement are immense. By liberating vata, we can increase feeling to make change in the form, which in turn can enable change in the self-image. When the self-image is changed, the learning is more complete and the change is well-established.

Let's look at Mike's troublesome knee joint. Possibly due to some trauma, the membranes around his knee became shrink-wrapped, thickened and congested, like putting plastic around an item and applying heat. "Shoop" and it's tight. The membranes got so tight and congested that they restricted the flow of vata. The air was squeezed out from stagnation and lack of movement. It became necessary to break up the congestion manually, using a tamasic touch vigorous deep contact, a direct approach to free the movement and enliven the nerves. If we are to find the healing memories within the tissues of Mike's knee, we must reclaim it in the self-image. For us to help Mike re-incorporate the knee as part of himself, he must be able to perceive it, to feel it. For that to happen, we need to release the vata. Vata is the only mobile component which transmits a sense of touch to the brain and other parts of the body. It's that electrical stuff zooming through the body going, "Oh, I just stepped on something sharp" quickly enough so that we can get off before it penetrates our skin. Thank God for the quickness of vata. The direct touch (tamasic) can break up the congestion, increase movement, and release the ability to feel. Once we are able to feel ourselves clearly through the balanced movement of vata, we can better manage the other elements. Having adequate power to move and feel through healthy vata, we can mobilize the water and earth of our kapha. We can send water to cool the excessive fire, or fan the fire with the air of the free-flowing vata principle.

I was in Alaska, working on a client's abdomen, and I noticed something starting to happen under my hands. I thought, "Well, you know, I'm not invading here, so I'll just follow until it unwinds and see what happens." She felt better. I got a call from her a week or so after I returned to New Mexico. "My ovarian cyst went away." I didn't know she had one. The point is, there isn't a bolt of lightning that I shot in there and healed her, but the membrane restriction that may have held that pocket of material in a cyst-like form was given enough slack and enough fluid to unwind itself. The membranes, perceiving a safe non-threatening touch, released the healing memory of the flesh. The capsule of the cyst contained the knowledge of how to unwind itself. With a combination of just following and listening, and some knowledge of organ position and where to go next, together we worked the combination that unlocked the cyst.

Later a guy I had worked on in Alaska called up and said, "Hey, two days after you left I released a whole mess of gallstones." I didn't know he had a gall bladder problem. This is the nature of the work. Listen well, follow, and pay attention to where you are in the living book, and often good things happen.

INTERVENTION USING THE TOUCH OF AWAKENING

Information enters the nervous system as news of a difference.
-Moshe Feldenkrais

The Touch of Awakening points out in a physical way our existing needs which might have been neglected for a period of time. We get into a pressure situation and decide, no matter what, we have to keep going. We wake up and our body is clearly saying, "Don't do it, man. I'm telling you I'm on the edge. If you go to work, we're surely going to get ill." And we go, "Hey! It's 6:35. I'm getting up." We forge ahead, ignoring an existing need. The body will put up with that for a while. It's sort of like the oxygen debt: we run fast for a long distance and afterwards we're wheezing until our body catches up to its normal oxygenation and decarbonizes.

But these existing needs don't go away. They're registered somewhere in our body: in the soft tissues, in the immune system, in the adrenals, in the emotions, and encapsulated as life impressions in the membranes. When we wall off experiences and store them in our bodies for future reference, the membranes become tenacious enough to separate the local area from the rest of the system. The area is not part of the communications network; it's cut off from support and safety. If we have sustained a trauma, the tissues laminate so we can't feel the area, we separate from the pain, protect ourselves. If this lasts for too long a time, it becomes habitual and we lose this area in our self-image. Functionally, as life goes on, it becomes very important to have that area be accessible. We need that knee; we need those genitals. We want and need to feel like a whole being.

To reclaim whatever parts have been estranged, we start to look for a way around the walls, around the inhibitions, a way to feel again that open childlike sense. We need to build conscious bridges to the lost islands of our organism. We need intervention. For this, the Touch of Awakening is ideal. The Touch of Awakening begins the process of personal healing through understanding, and releases the information held in the tissues. Intervention through the Touch of Awakening increases awareness, safety, and support to such a high degree that we gain access to the space between our environments, or we might say we become aware of ourselves in neutral, a place from which we have more choice in our actions. Having some awareness of ourselves in the neutral space, we can use ourselves more efficiently and clearly. We can connect our random movements and parts of ourselves to function again as a whole being.

To more or less quote Moshe Feldenkrais: "If you can do something, you can undo it." If you're always blowing out your knees and ankles because they are so thin and you've got this big pyramid-type structure up on top, you can unmake it, or soften it. At the very least you can peek into what the structure is good for and learn what to do when it gets in the way. With the addition of information released with the touch response, you can begin to understand why and how you shaped yourself in such a manner, and thus have what you need to improve and make choices. If you're stuck with any kind of beliefs, or patterns of acting, it's going to be a troublesome life. We want options.

The Touch of Awakening is a tool that can help you increase or decrease the attributes necessary for making change. This is not about the therapist doing something to or for the client. This is simply being here, listening. What the touch generates can be profound. We need add nothing but love and caring.

In all the treatments that follow, we start out with the Touch of Awakening. Try the exercises. Get a partner and explore. Read the exercises to one another, or make a tape and listen to the exercises from your own voice. Do not limit this work to a therapeutic situation; this is for life as you find it, any daily event. The following exercises can help us in awakening and assisting others in their own transitions.

HOW TO INTERVENE

Using the Touch of Awakening

(1) Increase curiosity. Listen with your hands and soften your eyes. You are not looking for what is wrong; you are looking for what is there. Be neutral in your observation. Note the positions, rhythms, and general state of the client's being. "Hum. What is this in front of me? How curious that the head is slightly rotated." Try not to come to any conclusions; just stay in curiosity mode. At the beginning of any treatment, at the beginning of each stroke, empty yourself and simply observe.

(2) Make contact. Sit with your client or partner. It doesn't take a big procedure or a whole lot of ceremony, just simple acknowledgment that there's something special about us being here together. We have some time to spend together; this could be profound. At the current neutral position, very slowly and delicately make physical contact. Feel your way into the physical body. You must travel through the energy body and be given access to go further into the form. Take the time necessary to gain permission.

You are joining two nervous systems, two electrical systems and two physical systems. If you have an agenda, on the initial contact, you shut down the current because your mind is busy thinking and there's less potential for natural expression and awakening. The other body cannot be free to speak if your agenda is talking. Be quiet. Techniques will work because of the relationship that you establish person-to-person at this initial contact phase of the interaction, not because of the particular technique itself.

(3) Listen. This is a tactile listening. Listen for movements of fluid underneath the surface of the skin, movements of the layers of the tissue, changes in temperature, changes in vibration of the energy, the pulse, the rhythms they are expressing. Your listening has an amplifying effect on the changes that are transpiring; you become a sounding board for their self-corrections.

When you settle in ever so slightly, the vata response to touch is awakened, heat is generated naturally between your hand and the pitta just under the recipients skin; congested kapha melts, and any number of other experiences and elemental changes may transpire.

As the kapha between those layers begins to liquefy, the strain that's involved in the layer begins to reveal itself. There are potential strain factors held in place which may be counterbalanced by the soft tissue gristle. As the gristle yields to one's touch, that which is under strain starts to release. It's the Jack-in-the-Box principle: if the constraints are released, out comes Jack.

As you rest your hand on your client's body, with no intention, energies transpire and safety accumulates. "Wow, that feels good. He or she is not going to do anything to me that I wouldn't like." With that thought alone, more awareness and more safety accumulate. The feeling of safety adds to the biochemical changes initiated through the non-invasive touch and soon the client's body is yielding, its pattern of strain-contained energies is freed, and the healing memories are set in motion.

(4) Follow that drift. After the responses have taken place, the safety has increased, the elements have started some transition, and the understanding of how to be free is emerging (another way to think of the healing memories), there will be physical actions occurring under your hand. Sometimes this is very subtle, like a lump of butter beginning to slide across a hot skillet. Other times larger movements are forthcoming. Whatever happens, follow as precisely as you can. Don't push or lag behind, and stop when the movement stops. This passive assistance again amplifies the signal that is being given by the body, and again the recipients can better read their own living book..

(5) First intervention. After you follow the initial response for a short distance, you'll feel a natural place where it slows down or stops. At this point, you're on the edge of the self-image, the person's boundary. At this place we are often blind in our self-perception; this is generally where we stop learning, exploring, and growing a delicate place, but rich for making change. We now intervene by taking them a little farther in the same direction they were going. This action really gets the attention. The fact that your contact is there and offering support, coupled with the fact that you have slightly exaggerated a familiar pattern, makes them willing to risk a look. This edge is where some of the biggest change can take place in our lives.

The exaggeration slightly tips the scales, which brings the recipients balance into a new relationship (in essence, they are in a different relationship with themselves). They've followed this, and all of a sudden they're here at the edge and into a new place. "Wow! I didn't know it was that far over. Let me fix that." And they begin self-correction; the brain and nervous system are set in motion to self-correct. It's as simple and complex as that, a simple touch with a great deal of intelligence to follow. Healing starts from that position neurologically, consciously, and elementally. All the wisdom that's stored in the organism begins to activate and self-correct or adapt to something new and wonderful.

(6) Follow the self-correction or return to neutral. After your exaggeration or intervention, you can feel the self-correction manifesting. Follow where that goes, then return to neutral. Get back to wherever the neutral might be and it might not be in the same place after you've done the first intervention. Remove your hand from the body, reinvestigate, return (if you have left) to the curiosity stage. Notice differences. This is where the real learning begins. While "nothing" is being done, much can be learned.

The Touch of Awakening can help liberate existing needs because, at least for a short while during meaningful contact, we have more support and the attention is focused. When our attention is focused and there is an increased level of support and safety, the existing needs, the historic imprints, can arise.

Historic imprints can go 'way back. Dr. Lad said the history of our past lives is etched in our bone. Normally, we don't remember our past lives because the memories would confuse us; we have enough drama going on in this life. Why bring in more, right? But sometimes, to resolve things that are going on in this life, these memories are helpful. On occasion, touching somebody can bring up those lost files, as well as instigate changes in the physical body. "Geez, now I understand why my back hurts every time I'm around this person because he hit me with a mace in the back when I was in Egypt... am I glad I got that fixed up!" It's gone. Resolved.

This way of thinking may be a little cosmic for some of you. Let me give a more grounded-in-this-life example. As the tissues of your chest begin to release and re-organize with the aid of touch, you may recall a time when you fell over the handlebars of your bike and hit your chest so hard all the air was knocked out. As you lay gasping on the ground, you thought, never again will I try that. From that time on you stayed away from anything that had the slightest amount of risk. In so doing, you had little excitement in your life. In treatment, your chest unravels and you take a giant breath. You decide it is possible to put some risk-taking into your life: that relationship

172

you have been putting on hold, the roller coaster ride you've always wanted to try. In short, a gentle touch brought about a new infusion of excitement and vitality.

Resolution can come from such a simple touch. By bringing up lost files, historically imprinted in our tissues and bones, we have a chance to look over the information and update the files. When we become aware of more support and safety in our system, we can look at our self-organized patterns. We can begin to see why we clamp down on our chest when certain subjects are spoken of, or when we are around certain people. When somebody touches our chest in a meaningful way, we can literally re-examine how we store the strain pattern and why.

In the following exercise we will investigate some of the skeletal connections from the sternum and integrate them through assisted movement and personal awakening. Everything is connected in the human form. Although we will be focusing on the sternum, there is a strong relationship to the heart from working with the chest. Take notice of the effects that you can have on the openness and ease about the heart through interaction with the bones and tissues of the chest and the consciousness they represent. Again, as we prepare for more involved treatments in the next section of the book, it is helpful to have a sense of your own heart space.

Exercise:

Working Underneath the Patterns

Using the TOA

Have your partner lie on the floor or massage table. Place your hand slowly on his sternum, the breast bone, right in the middle of the chest. Touch very gently, as if you were a water bug landing on the water. If you land too hard, your wings get wet and you're swept out to sea. Very, very gently. Rest there, listening. You're in the listening mode now. Close your eyes. Feel the structure move as the person breathes. Maybe it doesn't move very much. Be curious.

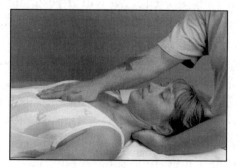

Do you notice a change under your hand? What is it? Does the sternum move upward, downward, sideways? What happens? On the next exhalation, follow where that bony structure goes. Ever so slightly, as your partner exhales, follow the movement.

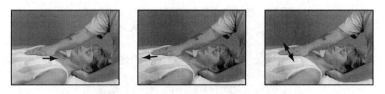

After following, exaggerate. Take it just a little bit farther in the direction you thought it went. Hold there. Now release. You're still on the body, but you're no longer following or exaggerating. You're back to wherever neutral is and you're listening again.

Make contact again. This time, examine if that region slides more easily to the right or to the left. Now you're intervening just slightly. Test it. If you push slightly to the left and then slightly to the right, which way does it go most easily? Choose the easiest direction. Lean that area toward that direction. This feeds information back to the nervous system about what the body does well. It's like a touch-release cabinet door: push it in and it comes out; try to pull it out, it doesn't do anything.

Release back to neutral. Meanwhile, recipient, take a breath or two. Notice how you're feeling. Be curious about these things and, absolutely, if anything being done is inappropriate, painful or what-have-you, please tell your partner.

Using very small movements, examine gently if the sternal region slides more easily upward toward the chin or downward toward the pelvis. Based on what you think you've found, take the person in that direction. Gently, using the following-then-exaggerating technique. Just a little bit farther than he's accustomed to, then back to center.

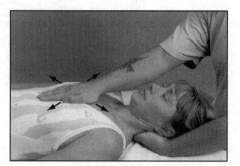

Slowly ease your hand off the body. Those who received the work, notice what happens when you breathe. Has something changed? With any luck, your partner hasn't imposed herself on you, just helped you do what you needed to do; so if you're feeling different, it's your own "fault".

Back to the same spot with one hand on the sternum. This time explore the diagonal glide. Ease the sternum diagonally downward and toward the opposite hip, then do the same in the other direction. Determine which direction the sternum moves most easily, then choose that direction, follow, exaggerate, and release to neutral.

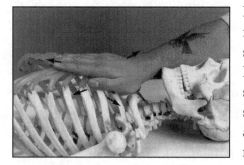

Now explore the same movement to the opposite diagonal. Again, follow gently, and at the stopping point very slightly exaggerate, hold a moment, then return to neutral.

Remove your hand from the body and observe. Recipient, breathe and feel your body. Note any differences. Don't limit your observations only to the sternum area. Scan your entire body for changes.

Place your hand again on the sternum. This time explore the opposite diagonal. Ease the sternum upward and to the left shoulder, back to center, then try to ease it toward the right shoulder. Choose whichever is easier and go in that direction first. Follow to the stopping point, wait, very slightly exaggerate, wait, then return to neutral. Rest a moment at neutral, then explore the opposite direction in the same gentle curious manner. Return to neutral and take your hand away.

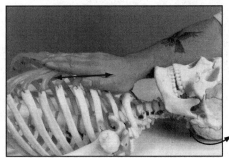

Integrate with pelvic movement

Observe and note differences. Recipient, begin to rock the pelvis upward and downward very slightly in order to include the sternum in the pelvic movement. Include the head. This will integrate the work you have received. Get up slowly and walk, noticing differences.

You may note a different feel, maybe an easiness in the chest, and possibly more connection to your heart. The next exercise helps clear the way for that heart energy to move into your world through your arms. We are not going to project something from our heart to the world or into the treatments, we just want that channel open to be able to feel and listen better through the environments and with other people.

Exercise:

Search and Rescue: Part I

Reconnecting the Arms to the Whole of You

We can search out and rescue those limited parts of ourselves. Lie on your back and realize there's absolutely nothing you have to do. Thank God. Have as much ease in your body, in your mind, as you can permit.

Notice how the floor contacts your back. Does the floor seem hard in certain places? Does it seem like it's yielding in other places? Maybe certain parts of your body feel really supported and other parts seem antagonized by that hard floor.

Notice how your limbs rest on the floor, particularly your arms. Are the palms out, upward facing, downward facing? Are they partially inward, maybe facing your hips? Just be curious. There is no right way. However they lie is right for you at the moment. Notice how your shoulders rest on the floor. Does one seem lower against the floor than the other? Is there more pressure on one scapula, one shoulder blade, than the other?

As gracefully as you can, roll to your right side. Place your left hand fist down in front of you. Find a comfortable place for that fist. If you need something for your head, make a pillow out of your right arm, or get a pillow and use it.

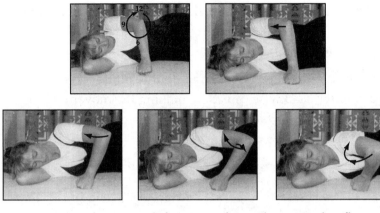

Keep the downward fist rooted in place on the floor. Imagine there's a circumference of eight or ten inches and you want to keep your elbow right in that circle. Explore making a clockwise half-circle about that circumference with your bent elbow. You are moving around the planted hand with your elbow in the air above it. Reverse the half-circle. Repeat this many times, then rest on your side with the arm relaxed.

Come back to the same position. Explore doing a three-quarter clockwise circle, and return several times. Note as the circle gets bigger which parts of your body are moving. Is it just the arm, or are you including the shoulder girdle and the ribs? Rest again with the arm relaxed on your side.

Return to the same position. Explore a full clockwise circle, slowly and gently. Your hand may need to roll over, so permit your wrist and hand to be soft enough to allow this to happen. Slowly continue making small circles and rest when you need to. Notice what your ribs are doing. Allow the spine to be pliable so that you can really flow with the elbow leading the movement.

Rest on your back. Notice how your arms are resting now compared to their original position. Move them gently and compare the ease.

Come up on the same side and do the same procedure in a counter-clockwise direction, making the movements as easy and comfortable as you can. Rest regularly, then lie on your back and compare differences.

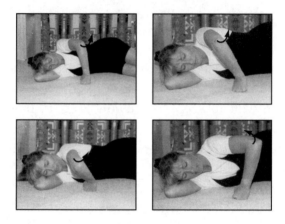

Variations in how we do things is often the most profound way to make change. I had an instructor in a Feldenkrais training who claimed to have shaved his face differently every day of his life. I can't imagine that. After a while you start running out of options. But every one of those options holding the hand this way or that works different neurological pathways in the brain.

To do a simple thing differently every time is a profound learning experience. Find something that you do habitually chewing your food on one side of your mouth all the time, reaching for a door handle with the same hand all the time, stepping into the car a certain way. Do it a little differently. See what you notice.

One way to define health is an ability to make change. Bodies can be vastly different in shape and yet may be very, very healthy. It's not so much a matter of how they shape themselves, but a question of whether or not they can learn. Can they make changes? As we do these simple exercises, we're softening our boundaries, softening the hard edge of habit in our minds. These exercises and Touch of Awakening practices are not only about the body, they're about the mind in the body.

Exercise:

Search and Rescue, Part II

Let's do the other side. Lie on your back. As you're lying there, imagine that your left arm is like the corn starch (see Corn starch exercise, page 117) that had been stirred up nicely, that all the lumps in the left side of your corn starch body have begun to melt and can ooze. Let the ooze transmit all the way through your body to the right arm.

Erase the boundaries of mechanics. You're an envelope containing five elements and consciousness in a liquid state. This is a truer representation of who you are than the hard anatomical model, so let yourself ooze from side to side, from top to bottom. Rock your feet up and down, so you're flexing and extending. Toes up toward your head and then down, several times rapidly. See if you can get the rest of your body to rock from the subtle, generated movement of your ankles. See if you can feel it coming through your head. Rock your own corn starch.

Let us begin with just the image of ourselves making the movements. Do these only in the imagination first. If what you want to do is not in the image, it cannot be done.

Roll onto your left side. Make yourself comfortable. Place your right fist on the floor in front of you. Imagine the circumference of a widening circle up to your bent elbow that's your constraint. Imagine making a clockwise half-circle with your elbow around your hand. Do it slowly enough so that all parts have a chance to participate in your mind. Notice, in your imagination, how your hip can be participating in this.

How does your spine participate in this activity? Feel free not to do this but to imagine it. How would you participate? How would your spine move? How would your vertebrae rotate? Now increase in your image to a three-quarter circle clockwise. Then do the whole circle. Be as clear as you can. See the spots that might be left out of the movement.

Now physically do the entire circle slowly 3 or 4 times. Does this fit with how you imagined it? Rest on your back, notice changes. Come back onto your left side and go through the same imagining process counter-clockwise, and finish with just 3 or 4 whole circles physically.

INTERVENTION

Any meaningful action done with an increase of safety and support will have far-reaching effects in creating lasting changes and options. The inverse is also true. Actions that are lacking in meaning and destructive in support and safety will inhibit your changes and restrict your options. The following story shows how attitude can get in the way of useful assistance in this work.

Many years ago, just after I graduated from massage school in Boulder, Colorado, I heard about John Fire Lame Deer, an Indian medicine man who was in the hospital in Denver, just an hour away. Paul, a friend of mine, came to me one day and said, "Do you want to go see John?" Having all sorts of fantasies about some magical man, a holy man, a healer, I was anxious to meet him, but really had no idea what to expect. Somewhere in the back of my mind, my ego began a drama. I had spent some years in training (studying acupressure and other modalities besides my massage background) and I was ready to heal the world. Why not heal the medicine man?

Paul and I drove to Denver. I was very excited, looking forward to "helping" John, who we found lying in the hospital bed with the most intense look, his eyes seemed to see into another realm. He had had a tracheotomy, so he couldn't speak, but that did not stop the communication. Paul sat down at the side of the bed and was just hanging out. Not knowing what to do, I pulled up a chair at the foot of the bed. Soon the therapeutic ego took charge. I held his feet, planning to give him a little energy. I found out later that if he had not wanted me to touch him, he could have prevented me from doing so.

As I was holding John's feet with all the love and caring I could muster, I looked into his eyes. The whole room, except for his eyes, became like the sky at night, with those little specks that seem to float in your vision. Then a voice came into my inner ear: "Who's healing whom?" I got the message. As I look back at this experience, I know I was not intervening, I was invading. Despite my good intentions, I was an intruder, and received a reprimand and a great lesson.

Be with the person and listen, wait to hear from their wisdom. Don't begin any treatment with an agenda. Even if we are right about what may need to happen, we must first consider who is doing the healing and who is in need of healing. I can't tell you how many times I have received great personal relief while working on someone. When we open the door of awareness and healing energy, and put no qualifications on it, there is a great wisdom that intercedes. So before applying technique, listen, follow, exaggerate, then begin to "lead" the awakening structure, belief and functional pattern into a new potential. And keep in mind who's healing whom!

It's like buying an upgrade or a new program for a computer. You put the information in your computer and then it says you need to reboot before this program will actually work. The same thing is true with this kind of bodywork. What we did while fiddling around wasn't nearly as important as the few moments afterwards of resting the time when your body absorbs the information before rebooting. When you turn off, it signifies to your body that all those changes have transpired; when you turn on again, your body can now use those changes. As we prepare to do more treatment work, remember the value of resting in neutral.

SECTION III

Treatments and Resources

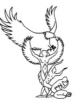

Chapter Eight

Vital Air Treatments

Settling a dispute between two students, the Master said, "Mankind has only one real enemy ignorance. Let us work together for its destruction, helping and cheering one another along the way."

- Paramahansa Yogananda

In the development of Life Impressions work, I have found that it is not enough to throw a number of techniques together and assume everything will come out all right. I put Life Impressions work under close scrutiny. First, the work must apply to the individual patients and their ability to utilize the work. Even if you have confidence in your process, the process must be made to fit the needs of the recipient. I have found the Life Impressions process must change with each new patient, and the manner of treatment must change with the time of year. The patient's individual constitution, as based on Ayurvedic principles, must be considered next. Finally, the work must be offered with awareness, safety and support. With proper attention to these factors, the treatments will have a much better chance of being helpful.

The treatments offered in this section of the book provide some subtle intervention or direct techniques. It is not within the scope of this book to offer great detail on direct work, which requires supervision and training (available through the Life Impressions Institute and other qualified teaching facilities). Because direct intervention treatment may be very delicate, and can even pose strong challenges to the recipient, here we will offer fairly basic release patterns which enable and enhance the indirect work. Whether direct or indirect, all the work that follows is designed to awaken the need for change, increase functional ability on all levels of existence, and educate. The treatments follow the basic laws of the human system mechanically, elementally, emotionally and spiritually so that all aspects of the system are supported and safe enough for healing to take place.

Hands-on work enhances what you have read in earlier portions of this book about personal awakening, safety, and support, the seven tissue layers and the components of the system, as well as the in-between states where the bio-chemical/elemental and emotional transitions occur, and makes it your own. The only true learning is that which is passed through our own experiential understanding.

It is important to note that "reversibility," a word often used in Feldenkrais movement therapy, is of great value. By reversibility we mean the ability to change directions at any given point in time with a minimum of effort, mentally or physically, to the advantage of the system. Reversibility can be impaired by our attitude; therefore we must have clear intention, but no personal agenda. There is great wisdom in the human organism, energetically and physically, particularly when working with these subtle vibrations. Although we will indicate a certain direction of flow and gently enhance that potential movement, we are in fact keeping the "reversibility potential" open for the recipient, and respecting any blocks he or she may have and still need. To offer an analogy: the recipient may need to back up with the energy and "make a run for it" as one would do on a snowy hillside. Listen carefully enough to allow for any such curious maneuver. As you become more proficient at offering treatments, your skill at staying out of the recipients path will be greater.

The treatments follow a particular order: building from pure spirit and thought, progressing into the tissue layers, and finally into the structural components of the complete human organism we inhabit every day. If we understand how this vehicle of ours is built, we can better understand how to fix it. If we consciously attend to each aspect of ourselves, we can discover the beliefs we impose on ourselves and the way they impose limitations on our functions and freedom in life.

It makes sense to start the treatments with the finest of the components in the body, the flow of the five vital airs. As we begin, please understand that although these energies are subtle, they are at the center of our very physical universe. The proper functioning of these profound forces may be the difference between vital health or just getting by on our reserves.

It is advisable to review the section on the five vital airs, consider their actions in the human form, and how they provide the power for more gross functions to be established and maintained. For example, an action supported by the vital air movements is the processing of information. Based on our choices and experiences, which may be stored in any number of places in the system, we respond to a stimulus. We may be inspired by viewing a spectacular sunset based on the movement of the energies in our system. The ability to feel the responses and process the insight or information is made possible by our energetic sponsors behind the scenes of the five vital airs. Much of the work we offer will have a greater potential for success if the vital airs are functioning clearly first.

Review the Touch of Awakening so you are well centered in the subtle, non-invasive aspect of the human touch. Remember, all this work is centered around awareness. If we lose that perspective, we are just going through the motions, pushing tissue around, rattling cages. The treatments are based on my experience and exploration using the concepts put forth in Ayurvedic material. I have seen great benefits result from these techniques, which are Western experiential applications based on 5000 years of study in the Ayurvedic medicine tradition.

As you practice the treatments, keep in mind the functions governed by each vital force. You may want to use these various treatments for specific ailments, either by themselves or in conjunction with other work. For instance, if there is sluggish elimination, try the apana treatment. Joint stiffness may be helped with vyana, and so on. Because we are dealing with a vital air, it can be helpful to apply warm oil on the area after you work to supplement the treatment and stabilize the vata.

A Reminder About The Three Types of Touch

Tamasic a strong contact, used primarily in direct work to break up congestion, re-establish contact with isolated parts. It can get the attention, melt the collagen from the old life impressions hardened through time, disuse, or overuse. Tamasic touch increases the flow of vata.

Rajasic a vigorous to gentle rocking, used to 'stir up the pot,' to mix up components and expand them into something more integrated and complex.

Sattvic light gentle touch of balance, sometimes known as spiritual touch. Sattvic touch takes us deeper than the tamasic, creating interest in the brain and nervous system.

It is said that one must gain conscious control over the life-force, breath, and mind to enter the deeper states of consciousness. By increasing our awareness of the subtle inner energies, as well as by establishing a clear directional flow of these energies, we can improve the control of our life-force for both our inner search for spirit and the well-being of the body and mind. This requires a great deal of inner attention and profound focus; one of the reasons why, for thousands of years, the saints and sages have taught meditation techniques, including pranayama (breathing techniques). May these treatments aid your well-being on all levels.

THE PRANIC CURRENT

Treatment of the Five Vital Airs

Imagine the prana (the life-force) as a soft, profoundly intelligent globe of energy within the crown of the head. When flowing naturally, this energy can be used either to enhance or reduce the activity of the senses, such as bringing vitality to tired eyes or more clarity to the auditory sense. This requires deep concentration and practice in meditation. In daily life, while we are functioning in the world, the pranic energy would prefer to move downward toward the lungs and heart; during sleep and deeper states of meditation, we want this energy to move upward to the crown. Awareness of this pranic current is the key to moving it in the most helpful direction for any given situation.

In your mind's eye, picture the flow of this vital energy moving downward to nourish the sense organs in the head and the lungs.

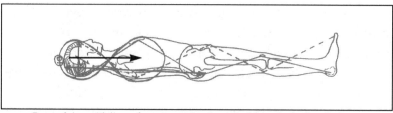

Person lying with lines of energy moving downward from the head to the lungs

Proper movement of this current can enhance the functioning of all the senses, energize the lungs, provide energy for the heart and ground the individual by anchoring consciousness in the body.

Treatment for The Pranic Current

Have the recipient lie on her back with eyes closed.

Make contact with your left hand on the top of the head, very softly, as if touching a sleeping baby. Listen. Wait to feel any response, such as a spontaneous breath or some subtle movement of the bones of the skull under your hand, or a sense of building awareness of the energy present in this area. See or feel the globe of vitality (you may find it of value for the recipient and yourself to imagine the energy in the region). Place the right index finger and thumb next to your left hand thumb side.

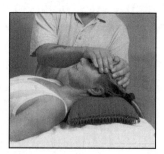 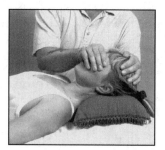

Wait for any response. On the recipients inhalation, as the diaphragm descends, begin to glide downward with the right hand, following the natural downward flow of energy. Stop at the end of the inhalation and wait for the next inspiration. This gets the recipient and yourself in tune with the dynamics of the breath. As you move down, stop at the corners of the eyes and wait for the energy to "soak in." Stay there for a breath or two while your awakening touch enhances the penetrating aspect of the pranic current into the eyes.

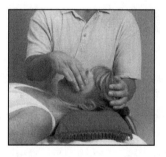 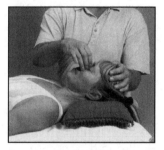

With the next breath, continue to move the right hand down to the sides of the bridge of the nose and rest there gently. Wait for a breath, again enhancing the pranic current. Have the recipient breathe "it" in. Gently glide down the 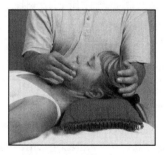 cheeks to the corners of the mouth, the index finger on one side, the thumb on the other, and rest there for a breath or two.

During the entire procedure keep in mind the downward moving current of energy, and let the left hand remain on the crown of the head. Let the right index finger move on the inhalation to the left ear, and place it gently into the ear opening. Wait for a breath.

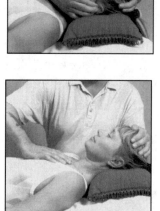

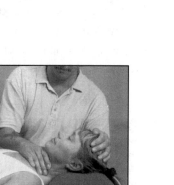

Place the right hand gently on the throat, and ride the inhalation down to the area where the bronchi split. Wait there for another breath, then again using the thumb and index finger, track outward and downward to the lungs. Wait again for the energy to settle into the area. Finally settle over the heart, letting the prana nurture the heart (prana must be available for vyana to function.) Once the hand is resting on the heart, imagine you are receiving the prana into the site of vyana. Imagine the spiraling action of vyana beginning.

After the prana treatment, have the recipient slowly rise and walk around; explore the differences.

THE VYANA CURRENT

Imagine a rotating globe of vitality within the heart, with the power to move all the fluids in the human body through the many miles of vessels. Proper circular movement of the vyana current can enhance the circulation of all fluids, the functions of the heart, and the circular motions of the joints. See this energy swirling outward from the dynamo of the heart region, adding spirals and circles to movement in life. Excess fire tends to shut down the feelings of the heart; in like fashion, movements may become mechanical, linear. The flow of vyana is needed. Even to imagine a circular action, prana and vyana must be present and active first the vital life-force, then the image or thought, and finally the action.

Treatment for The Vyana Current

Vyana cannot operate without prana, therefore begin with the left hand on the crown, enhancing the awareness of the pranic current. Place the right hand over the heart very gently, with great care and curiosity.

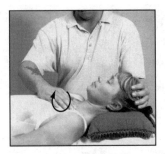 Imagine your hand being magnetized by the inner energetic movements coming from the heart. Feel the connection of the prana joining with the force of the spiral in the heart area. You may note the throbbing of the heart. Imagine with each pump of the heart the circular motions of the blood as it is moved along in the body. Subtly let your right hand begin to emulate the clockwise movement under it, beginning with very small movements. Like the center of

a gentle tornado, feel the winds extending outward from the eye of the storm. As the edges of the storm extend outward, the structures that are touched can also move with the circular pattern.

Keeping your right hand over the heart area, now move your left hand down and place it on the left shoulder (a structure that needs efficient circular movement) and begin to move the hand on the shoulder in harmony with the one on the chest.

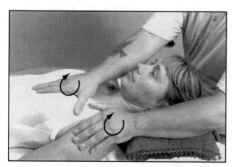

Continue to move in the circular pattern for several revolutions. Please note you are enhancing the energetic potential for physical movement, not creating movement on a gross level. This action should be very gentle, hinting at the potential that the energy can provide.

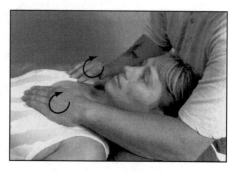

Now move your right hand to the right shoulder and enhance the circular potential, always keeping one hand over the heart. (As you contact other areas you may have to switch hands.) Offer several revolutions at the right shoulder; move on to the left hip, then the right. Choose any place that you perceive to be in need of rotational awareness, the ribs, ankles, the neck, joints of the finger, and enhance there.

This technique can be offered with the person on his stomach if need be to accommodate other areas, such as the subtle rotations of the vertebra and sacrum. As you did on the front of the body, place the hand on the area of the heart on the back, the other hand on the crown of the head, and then proceed as you did on the front to the areas in need.

After the vyana treatment, have the recipient slowly rise and walk around; explore the difference.

THE UDANA CURRENT

Through its actions on the body and mind, the udana current is responsible for all upward movements. (I once thought about doing udana clinics for athletes, particularly basketball players.) Udana is responsible for many functions; even the idea of a certain action is not possible if this vital current is not available. One of the actions udana directly effects is memory; for the memory to work, the brain must receive information from the body. The ability to remember how to reproduce actions in the body, the functional memories, are particularly under the influence of udana. For example, in order to take the next step in walking, the energy containing the information about picking up the foot must be able to travel to the foot, which happens through the downward-assisted action of prana and apana, and return to the brain, via the upward mobilizing power of udana.

The blueprint pattern for the idea of an action is spawned by the vital energies; as the act occurs and is repeated, it becomes functionally etched in the brain grooves by recruiting some neurons for the pattern, and etched in the tissue by recruiting the fascial or membrane network and shaping itself to the task like gelatin hardening in a mold. The program is set in place. To repeat the pattern again, you must have the information activated by the vital airs before the nerve electrical response can act.

In the West, we have used microscopes and other aids to investigate and prove the smallest actions we can see, and still we are baffled by the brain and nervous system. It cannot be dissected or seen by normal means; this is something that must be felt. A few examples of the udana response which we often take for granted are the upward movement of the material in the ascending colon, opening the eyelids, lifting the head, and standing up. On a subtler level, raising the energy in meditation and leaving the body at the time of death are under the control of udana.

Treatment for the Udana Current

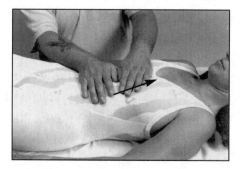

Have the recipient lying on his back, with the practitioner sitting on the right side of the table. Imagine the subtle vitality that sustains all upward movement building under the diaphragm, a great potential for vertical extension, resting and ready for use. Place your right hand on the body just below the rib cage. See if you can feel that potential energy for upward thrust; this is the main area where udana is stored.

Begin to feel and follow the breathing as the chest and lungs fill with breath, the diaphragm is descending; as the chest and lungs empty, the diaphragm is ascending. (In truth it is udana that is arising. That in turn elevates the diaphragm.) It is on the ascending action of the diaphragm that the udana can be enhanced. As the diaphragm rises slightly, enhance the movement.

Place the right hand on the ribs just below the left hand. (Although we are enhancing and following the breath, do not lose sight of the fact that it is this subtle energy we are attuning to, not the breath. It is just a physical vehicle.) After you enhance the upward flow using the diaphragm, which in essence enhances the flow of the upward udana current, "catch" the flowing energy with the left hand and carry it up the front of the torso.

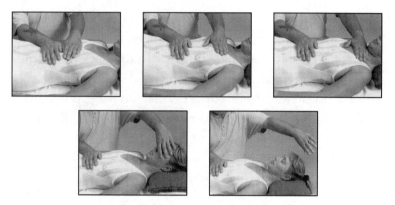

Continue this action with the hands, carrying the energy to all areas of the torso arms, head and so on anywhere you feel the need to have a sense of lift. (Wait at each area for a moment to mentally "fill in" the space where your hand rests.)

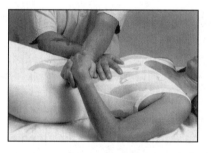

Place your left hand on the arch of the recipient's left hand. Follow the rhythm and exaggerate upward, then brush the vitality upward along the wrist, forearm, and upper arm. Do the same with the arch of the right hand.

A word about structure: if you put the feet together, the combined arches create another functional diaphragm. We might include the arches of the hands and the armpits as functional diaphragms as well. All these arched structures behave functionally as diaphragms. For example, when the weight is lifted from the foot, the suspension membranes (the tissues on the bottom of the foot) recoil, providing an upward thrust like that of the diaphragm. The same pumping action takes place, subtly, even when these structures are at rest.

Try this: lie on your back and begin to slowly open and close your hands, while very gently flexing and extending the arch of the feet. Make this movement smaller and smaller until you totally leave it alone. Now feel the fluid and energetic actions continue on their own. In short, all the arches in the body are like pumping stations for the udana current. More to the point, udana pumps them and their action enhances the power of the pump.

Place your right hand on the arches of feet. Feel the potential vitality there; feel that subtle pulse that expands and then contracts as the energy and fluids are moved about in the area. If you cannot feel this pulse, then watch and co-ordinate with the breath: on the exhalation subtly press into the arch, enhancing the upward flow of udana.

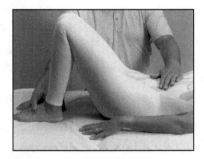

After the udana treatment, have the recipient slowly rise and walk around; explore the differences.

THE SAMANA CURRENT

The samana current of vital energy, primarily stored in the area of the small intestine, controls all linear movement. The lateral aspects of the spiral movements in human locomotion are under the control of this current of energy. Shifting weight from one foot to the other while walking requires samana, moving the food in the intestines from side to side requires samana, transmitting information between the two hemispheres of the brain requires samana, and so on. To reconstitute these actions physically is very difficult; it can be made easier if you first establish the flow of the samana current for linear action, then the awareness of the movement possibilities that arise from lateral potential can be put into action. This energy has a great deal to do with our ability to digest or process what we receive as nourishment. My feeling and personal experience is that this translates not just to the digestion of food but also to ideas and actions.

Treatment for the Samana Current

Recipient on back; practitioner sitting at the right side of the table. Place the left hand on the area between the navel and the area of the small intestine, the storage area for samana energy. Imagine vitality flowing from side to side under your hand.

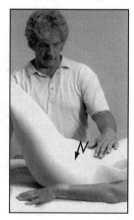

Begin to follow it gently. If you cannot feel it, just begin to slightly shift your hand from side to side. Your physical movements will enhance the vital energetic, and vice versa.

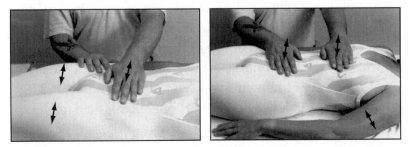

After you have awakened the samana in the lower abdomen, place your right hand on the right side of the pelvis and begin to rock it in concert with the one on the abdomen. Then, sliding your left hand up to the rib cage, continue the rocking and transfer the sense of vitality to that area. Go up to the shoulder and then the arm (the whole time continuing to rock at the abdomen), then include the leg.

Do the same on the left side. Have the recipient rest, then explore walking.

Note: You may slowly take the rocking movement down the legs and arms while keeping one hand on the abdomen.

THE APANA CURRENT

Apana, the downward current emanating from the lower pelvic cavity, is the governor for all motor functions for the pelvic cavity and its organs. This vital current is responsible for all elimination from the lower body, gas, urine, feces, fetus, sperm, and ovum. Virtually any downward action, including actions of the lower limbs, is controlled by apana.

The peristaltic action of the large intestine is under the control of this vital air, and can be easily disturbed by congestion, constipation or other colon problems. In Ayurvedic medicine, vata, the air and ether elements and one of the three main constituents of the human being has its main seat or container in the colon. Vata also controls the nervous system and the mind. We can readily see how this area can be compromised and lead to a nest of trouble when dysfunctional. Excess movement in the bowel will overflow energetically (a process called samprapti in the East and pathogenesis in the West) into the pelvic bones, interrupting nerve flow, joint function and spinal alignment. We may have back aches, sciatica, even excess neurological problems such as numbness or spasticity.

Apana, in my observation, is the vital air most often in disharmony. This observation is supported by the great number of unsolved back problems and the preponderant use of laxatives in our culture. Back problems and colon congestion can arise from injury, bad diet, poor functional activity, nervousness, emotional holding but regardless of the origin, apana must be re-established in its normal balance before complete recovery can be maintained. Other therapies may be needed, but without the sponsor the show will not go on.

Treatment for the Apana Current

Recipient lying on the back; practitioner at the right side. Place your right hand on the abdomen just above the pubic bone, and left hand parallel to the right (the pelvic diaphragm).

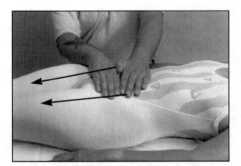

Begin to imagine the power of apana building, and magnetizing itself to the earth. Synchronize with the breath. The inhalation will cause the pelvic floor, another diaphragm, to descend toward the feet. Follow the subtle descent of the movement. (Do not move the hand over the body, just press very gently in the same direction.)

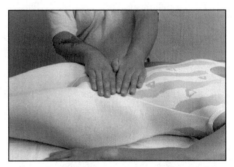

Place the right hand on the right leg at the top of the thigh. On the inhalation, move the enhanced flow of apana by brushing downward. Stop between breaths. Imagine the vitality building under your hand at that point, and then continue downward with the next inhalation to the sole of the foot.

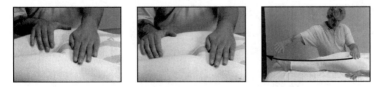

Then do the left leg in the same manner.

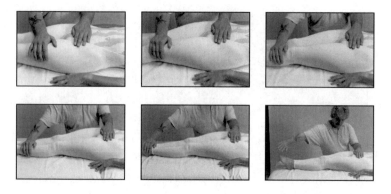

Contact the sole of the foot (another diaphragm) while maintaining the contact with the pelvic diaphragm. Synchronize the actions, keeping the image of the apana current in mind.

Have the recipient get up and walk around; note any differences.

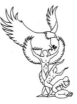

Chapter Nine

Component Treatments

There are many components that make up the human system: consciousness, the five elements, the membranes, the outriggers, the three cylinders, the girdles, and the inner membranes. The five vital air treatments from the previous chapter enhance the energetic wisdom and actions for all activities, enabling the recipient spiritually, energetically, emotionally, and physically. I encourage you to practice these treatments and offer them first in order to get the best results from any other treatment. It is not within the scope of this book to offer detailed treatments for all the components; some are better presented in other forms more technically oriented books, classes, videos, and audio tapes (available through the Life Impressions Institute).

There are very clear steps to be followed when working with some of the systems, particularly the tissue layers. When you interrupt the layering, there must be adequate support developed beforehand. The following treatments can build support, release self-organization, and enhance elemental balance. All the treatments are gentle and non-invasive, built around the organization of the elements, the dhatus, and the structural components of the human being, and should be of great value.

The membranes encase every component in the human organism and must be dealt with based on their potential dominance of any given structure. Although it is not appropriate to delve into great detail regarding membrane and structural intervention, it is necessary to tend to the membranes and at least "wake them up" for best results in treating the components. Having already done the five vital air treatments, you have accessed the consciousness and the five elements at a subtle but powerful level. To some degree, this also awakens the membranes, making them available for further work. To further the awakening, I have added a simple but very effective process called "sleeve release and integration," which softens the membranes' imprinted habitual patterning and loosens the constraints the membranes may impose on various components. Please offer the sleeve work before you treat any of the components.

From there, we move on to the outriggers. We will not separate the three cylinders because these layers are so intimately engaged they require a great deal more understanding and study before intervening. Here we will treat them as a single unit, thus retaining adequate support.

THE SLEEVE RELEASE AND INTEGRATION TECHNIQUE

The following procedure can be offered to any area of the body. If the principles are adhered to carefully, many positive responses will take place. There are many layers of tissue around any given structure; (see Illustration, page 110). all the layers are designed for safety and support, therefore they are ready to respond to a stimuli if it is perceived as safe, pleasant, supportive and so on. Each sleeve (layer of tissue) when healthy and responsive, is "floating" on a thin layer of fluid that separates it from the next layer. All sleeves are composed of awareness and the five elements. Each layer or sleeve tends to want to maintain some communication with the whole organism, and therefore has a relationship to all other layers. With these factors in mind, we offer this treatment with great respect, realizing that the membranous order that is currently in place has been established according to experiences, patterns, feelings and so on. Change in the established tissue layering pattern is only received and positively acted upon if there is no threat to the safety and support already assumed by the organism. In short, work with great sensitivity and respect. Don't get lost in the technique; it is all about consciousness, about interaction, a conversation layer to layer throughout the system.

For practice we will use the fingers and arms, as they are easily accessible and can always use some work. Please transfer the same procedure to other parts of the system, particularly as they respond to the component treatments to follow.

The positive actions of this treatment differentiation of the layers of the system can liberate both congestion and contained information, awaken forgotten functional pathways, which in turn invite other aspects of the system to unravel in a similar manner. With added support, you can venture into actions that are very liberating on a subtle level. The differentiated layers provide space for the interstitial fluids to take up residence, which in turn retain the functional space by keeping the layers slightly separated and lubricated.

The Sleeve Release Technique

Close your eyes. This will heighten the other senses, particularly that of touch. Gently grasp your entire right index finger with your left hand, and wrap it softly with the whole hand. Please note: The indication 1st and 2nd relates to which body part should be activated in what order.

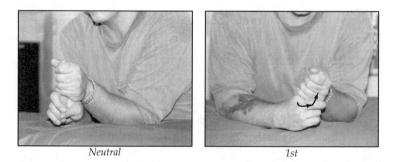

Neutral   *1st*

Using your right hand and finger, turn the index finger to the left very slightly, just enough to feel the bones move within the flesh, and wait there a moment. That lag time between this action and the next is essential for the physiological actions of fluid exchange and the awareness that permeates the system.

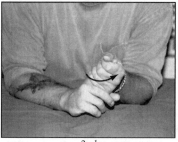

2nd

With the left hand, turn the sleeve of flesh about the finger to the left, just a small amount to become congruent with the bones. You are working only in the available slack space, the area of tissue bone differentiation that is currently available. Do not try to make more space! You are using the Touch of Awakening, not trying to make something change that will happen naturally with the increased awareness, safety and support.

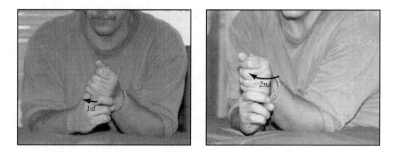

Turn the finger back to neutral, then bring the sleeve back to neutral. Explore the same pattern to the right, making sure to have enough time for a breath or two between the two actions.

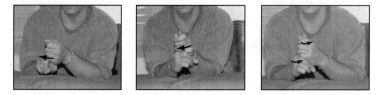

Repeat the same pattern but add elongation. For example, turn the finger to the left and slightly lengthen. After you match the pattern, turn back while shortening.

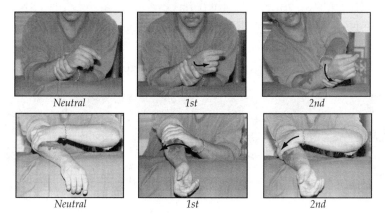

Neutral   1st   2nd

Neutral   1st   2nd

Try this with all the fingers, the wrist, the elbow, any body part that you can encapsulate without straining yourself to reach. Remember to move only a very small amount, move slowly, wait between bone movement and sleeve movement, rest and compare often. Become familiar with this sleeve technique on yourself, then practice on others. Finally, add it to the component work.

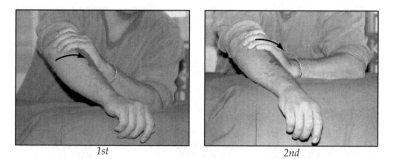

1st   *2nd*

THE OUTRIGGER TREATMENT

Review the section on the components of structure to familiarize yourself once again with the outrigger concept [page 138]. Think of stabilizers: imagine being on a tightrope with your hands at your side, then having your arms out with an extension pole for stabilization; imagine being on the high seas in a single-hulled craft or in a trimaran. This is the advantage of having our outrigger structures in place and functional.

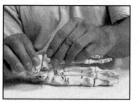
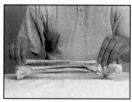
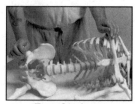

Foot   *Fibula*   *Torso Outriggers*

An anatomical review of the outrigger components includes: the outer arch of the foot, including the last two toes; the metatarsal, cuboid, and the calcaneus bones; the lateral bone of the lower leg, the fibula; the greater trochanter of the femur; the lateral aspect of the ribs; and the arms in general, the humerus. There are other structures that are pertinent to the lateral outrigger system, but they are not appropriate to offer in practical work through text alone; in following with the principle of safety and support, these others must be taught in a live class situation.

Prior to this treatment, please review and practice the Corn starch Exercise [page 117] in order to get into your hands the feeling of how the soft tissues and elements respond to touch.

The outrigger treatment structurally enhances the release and support of the other components, like peeling an onion while holding it. In the same manner, doing the sleeve work releases and increases the balance and support for the continued release of the outriggers. The outermost packaging creates room and support for the underlying structures to unfold. As we perceive and functionally experience a wider base, we can feel safer and trust that it is all right to open further.

Remember, as always, that we are not just structure, but in truth we are consciousness that has created a structure. With this in mind, think of the change in the relationship of the components as happening on all layers of tissues and throughout all aspects of consciousness at once, even though, for the sake of clarity, we talk about one component at a time and tend to focus our attention on one level of consciousness at a time. If you squeezed together many layers of compressed cellophane and then let go, all the layers would begin to unravel at once, although the top layer is most obviously in transition. Think of the Jiffy Pop popcorn gadget: you may only see the foil on top expanding, but the heat is expanding the kernels which in turn are expanding the top foil layer. We are not able to expand if the membranous sleeves (the popcorn) are glued together with congestion or with simple lack of use or awareness of movement potential. This missing dimension, the lack of differentiation, reduces fluid exchange and integration of larger movements. At the same time, it is awareness that is expanding under the widening outrigger, awareness in the sleeve tissues and throughout the system. The lag time we offer in the sleeve exercise permits the awareness to permeate, in essence giving us time to try the new feeling out, to learn a new way.

Realize that all the areas we will work with already know their proper relationship; that information is in our very make-up, it was in the design before we imprinted it or habituated ourselves. You need not make anything happen; the wisdom to clear the area in question is already in place, spring-loaded and waiting to be free. When we are assisting someone else, our job is to add support and safety, assist the spontaneous release, and guide the awakening. Don't get stuck in the anatomy. You are still working with awareness and the five elements, they just happen to be in a more concentrated form. Focus your attention on the area of potential change and get the recipient to meet you there; only then interact with the organism.

The information in this section is a prelude to the actual practice. There are details worthy of your consideration, but impossible to read while trying to practice. You want to be as free of mental ties as possible during practice so you can be with and listen to the person.

Outrigger Release Treatment

Have the recipient lie on her side with a small pillow under the head to keep continuity in the spine uninterrupted, and another pillow between the legs to reduce the strain on the hip joint. Have the knees comfortably bent to release strain on the lower back. With these simple details, you give signals to the nervous system to rest and relax, indicating to the system that it is safe, which will increase the ability for the nervous system to be available for learning and change.

Visualize the space between the two arches of the foot, the space between the 3rd and 4th metatarsals, putting your mind in the area where you intend to offer support. The first steps in transformation are awakening, increased support, and safety, which in turn increase the ability to explore new possibilities. By clarity of intention in visualizing, you begin to get congruent with the pattern in the human blueprint and thus assist the recipient in doing so.

Have the person slide close to the side of the table, with her back to you so that you don't have to extend too far and create strain in your own body. Your ease or tension can be perceived by the other person. Either standing or sitting, position yourself by the foot.

The Foot

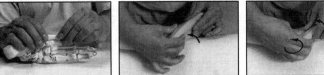
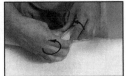

1st Client Movement　　　*2nd Practitioner Follow*

Sleeve release preparation: Gently place your hands parallel to one another, thumbs under the foot in the space between the 3rd and 4th metatarsal. Melt into the flesh. Let as much of your hand as possible make contact with the lateral foot. Have the recipient raise the lateral arch just enough to feel the bones move under the skin, hold there, wait, then ease the tissues upward to become congruent with the bones. Let the recipient return to neutral, then you bring the flesh back to neutral. The recipient rotates the lateral arch downward, waits, then you follow, wait. The recipient returns to neutral, and you bring the flesh to neutral. Now the area is better prepared for outrigger work. (Photo's, page 215)

Rest in that naturally occurring neutral space, using the Touch of Awakening. You are updating the blueprint. The body knows that there is a designed space under your fingers and will begin to enhance that space, with the assistance of the awakening touch. You are increasing air and ether (the elements in charge of the sense of touch, the mind and the nervous system). With the help of these mobilizing elements in the organism, old patterns can begin to move; inhibitions of habit anchored in the heavier elements can begin to release.

Wait for the meltdown, the transition of the heavier elements. Air and ether begin to fan the fire of intelligence, which ignites in the tissue spaces; the pre-molded earth and water patterns that make up the membranous sleeve begin to melt. You begin to feel the space between the bones, and the bones float apart in the more elastic membranous material.

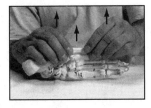 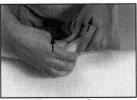

Separate arches

Gently begin tractioning upward (away from the rest of the foot) very slightly, with some rajasic movement (slight wiggling). You are creating some subtle suction; as the harder structures are widening, the interstitial fluids rush in to maintain the functional spacing. (Remember the practice of withdrawing something from the thick corn starch.) The entire arch system will begin to span at this point.

Hold at the full extension for a couple of breaths. In fact, direct the breaths into the space between the bones (the breath carries the attention; include this in all your work). The traction should be gentle. The foot should not rise off the pillow it is resting on. If it does, you are using too much traction.

In the short time that it takes to complete the stroke described, awareness penetrates the "new" space between the bones (the lower end of the membranous pathway), the interosseous membrane is accessed for movement transmission, and interstitial fluid rushes into the formerly dehydrated, laminated seam between the metatarsals. All this action permits the change to be well assimilated into the organic actions of the system. These factors, along with the awakening of the nervous system, enable the change to remain. In fact, now that the area has been hydrated, awakened, and the movement given a clear channel, it may well become the body's pattern of choice because of the ease with which it can be accessed.

Now that there has been some change in the outrigger system (at the very least more width and stability), begin to release the traction slowly; then rest in neutral while the system stabilizes. This completes the arch work for the outrigger treatment. (Although there is much more that can be offered, this is enough to practice.)

Compress the two arches together, following any spontaneous movements. For example, sometimes there will be a slight rotation or forward shifting of the bones. Include these as you perceive them, then gently slide the two arches against one another in a gentle sawing motion. Often compression satisfies the desire for a certain pattern of function that can then be re-educated or re-directed to be more suitable by the nervous system and the functional pattern in general. As you compress the congealed material, the deep dhatus in the core of the leg can be accessed.

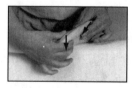 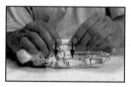

Repeat the above processes several times, then compare the differences.

The Lower Leg

Locate the fibula, the lateral bone of the lower leg. Gently palpate its entire length. (This introduces the nervous system to non-invasive touch and clarifies to the individual the personal image of the structure where it is, its contour, the part this structure plays in the system and basically heightens the self-image to include this part.) By differentiating the fibula/tibia junction, there is further clarification regarding the translation of movement through the interosseous membrane and the bones. The

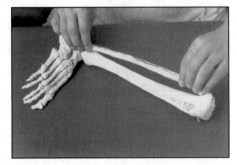

recipient gets a clear tactile sense of the support she has coming from the earth through the body, and exactly how it gets through the body. This is very valuable information and often taken for granted.

Grasp the two ends of the fibula and gently wiggle, then slowly pluck it from the underlying tissues. There is a physiological suction as the bone arises. Give adequate time for all actions to take place. The larger nerves and vessels rest in this space between the bones; as it becomes more available, the nourishment and sensory awareness is heightened, as well as the sense of support and transmission of weight from the ground up and down. Wait at the end of the traction. Again, have the recipient breathe into the area between the bones.

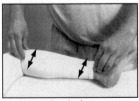

1st Action

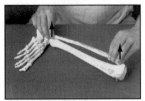

Pluck 2nd Action

Maintaining your grasp on the fibula, slide it up and down very slightly and rotate it forward and back.

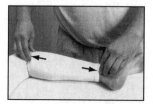 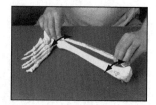

Stop, release the traction, and let the bone ease back to neutral. Let the recipient explore the differences. Compare the two feet and lower legs by gently moving them. The brain and nervous system learn by comparing differences.

Do the other leg; the very same procedure may be offered for the arms. Remember to make your movements very small. You may want to add some integration work, such as gentle massage to connect the limbs to the torso. At the very least have the recipient take a walk after this work to integrate it into the system further.

You as therapist may have two objectives: first, to assist the recipients in self-exploration and correction through awakening, establishing with them the support of their outrigger; secondly, to aid in clarifying the path of functional action through their structural maze.

The Ball-and-Socket Components

The four ball-and-sockets (shoulders and hips) provide pivotal actions for the limbs as well as "floating corners" for the pelvic and shoulder girdles. As far as those areas are concerned, the ball-and-sockets are their outriggers. As with the other outriggers, if they are wide and float gracefully on the surface of the joint capsule, they maintain a supportive flexible relationship to the inner components of the system. If there has been some compression in any of the ball-and-sockets, that compression in turn impairs the underlying structures and compromises that function. Because of the great flexibility of the ball-and-socket structures, they can enhance or impair function in many dimensions. The liberation of the ball-and-socket outriggers can be very beneficial to the entire system, enhancing the release of the lower outriggers as well as freeing the cylinders, the viscera, and the girdles.

You may think of the ball-and-socket as a floating organic parallelogram (a four-sided figure having equal and opposite sides, for those of you who were absent that day in geometry class). Any change in the length of one side requires some change in the three other sides. If you get smashed in the hip, the other three corners will have to change relationship relative to the impact, and/or the impact will have to be absorbed in the torso, which will in some manner reflect to the other corners indirectly. This treatment is designed to help the body restore the flexibility of the original parallelogram, and to share the load of any given imposition.

The Ball-and-Socket

Locate the greater trochanter and the greater tubercle (head) of the humerus (two of the four ball-and-socket structures).

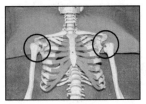 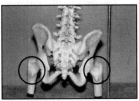

Sleeve prep:

Have the recipient lying on her side, supported as needed. Mold your hands to the hip and shoulder ball-and-sockets. Melt in for a moment. The recipient very subtly lifts the heel and elbow to rotate the bones foreward, and holds; the practitioner brings the tissues foreward also. The recipient comes back to rest in neutral, bringing the tissues back also. Repeat this a few times in both direction, then go on to the ball-and-socket outrigger release.

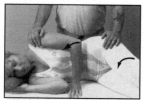

Heel & Elbow Movement 1st

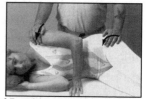

2nd Practitioner moves in same manner

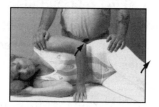

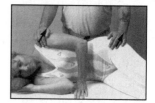

Remember that there is fluid surrounding all solid structures in the human organism. Even the solid structures themselves contain minute levels of fluid air and fire; they are not as solid as we imagine. The humeral head is literally floating on the synovial fluid underneath it, as is the head of the femur.

Make contact with the two ball-and-socket structures. Imagine you are grasping ping-pong balls in water. As you make contact, feel the viscosity under them and feel the ease of their glide. With one hand on both the humeral head and the greater trochanter (recipient lying on side) begin to very gently compress directly into the body; follow the squish in the direction that it prefers to go, then wait before going in another direction.

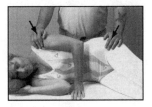 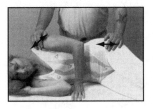

Explore other options minutely, 1/16 inch in various directions. This action serves to introduce options to a habit-bound system and clears the way so new patterns can be explored. After exploring several directions and waiting at each point, ease back to neutral and release your contact.

Grasp both bony heads of the humerus and the femur, gently and slowly traction upward and away from one another. Ease upward slowly about 1/4 inch, then wait for a couple of breaths. Slowly release the traction and encourage the two bones toward each other. Do this traction and release two or three times. Explore their forward (toward the front) movement as they are drawn toward one another, and then as you traction, spread the bones away and gently rotate them backward toward the recipients back. (See page 224)

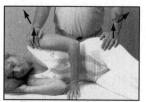
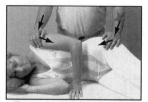

Traction upward & away   *Down & toward one another*

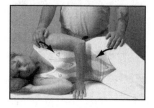
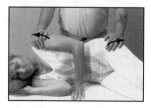

Have the recipient explore the differences side to side in a very gentle way. Complete the aforementioned steps on the other side. Then have the recipient take a walk around the room.

Before we go on, let us review for a moment our purpose in this work and gain a clear understanding of what may be offered with this treatment. We are first of all awakening and clarifying the functions of the elements and the components of the human system. We are continuing to enhance and utilize the five vital airs, which in turn enhance the functional aspects of the human system. We are increasing the clarity of the self-image and the ability to act with ease. Please do not allow these techniques to become mechanical for you. I encourage you to offer this work as information to enhance human potential for self-organization and self-learning.

If the recipients feel better, if problems are healed, let that be a by-product of their learning about themselves and the improved self-image they now maintain, not a mechanical fix they think you applied.

In any interactive therapy, one in which two or more persons are working together, it is important to remember integration, offering treatment work in a manner in which the person can assimilate and utilize it. In a sense, we create an environment for well-being and self-exploration. One of the integration factors, aside from appropriate contact, adding support and safety, listening and so on, is enhancing the felt sense the structural and energetic connection in the organism. By "felt sense" I mean kinesthetic awareness, not just the intellectual idea of the structures. This provides much information, both physically and neurologically, that the system can use for learning and self-organizing.

All organic matter (and even some that is inorganic) has a polar relationship, a magnetic quality including positive/negative and neutral energetic aspects. On a structural level, all organic matter has developed a top, bottom, and middle relative to its interaction with gravity and space in general, a kind of polarity in the physical area that it occupies. If the energy in the top of the body increases to a certain level, there is a need to dissipate or balance that vitality, which usually means taking it to the other end or moving it out of the system. It's like a straw: if you increase the energy by sucking on one end, the other end must respond or the straw will collapse, and possibly your cheeks will also collapse. But if the polarity or energy is balanced, the fluid moves and the integrity of the straw is intact. Assuming the energy is congruent with the system and usable in the organism, the energy would like to be shared with the rest of the system, equalized, unless there is a purpose for temporarily building a charge in some place. Even after we anchor to move something heavy, after that effort we want to bring the system back to energetic balance.

If we begin to move, we set in motion both energetic and physiological changes in the membranes and the skeletal and nervous systems, all of which require available translation potential to avoid blockages, spasticity or breaks in the continuity. With this in mind, while completing the outrigger treatment, we must continue by re-establishing the integration relative to the change in the organization of the system. We now need to clarify an under-structure and "poles" to enhance and further integrate the work we have been doing with the outriggers. The following portion of the treatment will enhance those factors.

At this point in the treatment, a more available and functional outrigger system has been awakened, although there is more to that system. Hopefully there has been adequate awakening and functional potential released, with the following results: more stability is erected as the "landing gear" or center of balance widens through the span of the outrigger components; more length and ease emerge as the lateral body parts are more fully able to widen; the main part of the body can afford to relax and release its contractions. When the main cylinder has the extra support of the functional outriggers, organizing the cargo is easier on digestion, fluid movements, and general physiology. If the large cylinder, the torso, has to be excessively aware of and participate too much in the struggle for balance, some of the functional energy is held in reserve for protection and may well affect the cargo handling.

Review the interplay between outrigger and main cylinders. The large cylinders are carried along with the outer layer opening and the main cylinder work. There is more specific work on all layers, but it is again not appropriate through text to try to convey such specifics. There is a natural tendency for the inner structures to begin to unfold as the outriggers are more available. In response to the outriggers being released, the deeper layers of tissue, the dhatus, are more available for functioning, cleansing, and circulating. With the main cylinder release, the structure becomes more stable, like raising the metal slide piece on an umbrella. There is better circulation of elements through all the layers, and communication to areas is restored.

This section of treatment can be done by itself, but will be better served if it follows the outrigger work. Please remember that these treatments are somewhat general; they can be applied to most people, if offered with respect and using the proper procedure. If you listen and follow carefully during treatment, you will inspire a very personalized experience for the person receiving the work; if you just follow the directions mechanically, it will be a mechanical treatment. There are certain limitations to what can be conveyed through the written word. I hope you will fill in the sensitivity, the compassion, and the personalization. If you use the principles of the Touch of Awakening, surely good things will happen.

Now back to the completion of the treatment. To set up the optimal qualities for polar balance and raise the main body mast, to free the core structures and spine, first we must be grounded; therefore we begin at the feet.

Integration of the Main Cylinder

Recipient on back, legs extended. Hold one foot, with one hand covering the inside arch, the other hand holding the outside arch. Your position alone enhances and clarifies the membranous space that passes between the two arches, through the bones of the foot, upward between the long bones of the lower leg, through the femur and deep membranes of the thigh, and emerges into the pelvic floor, sending sensory and structural messages upward and downward to and from the spine and torso.

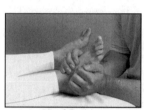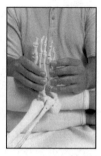

Hand Position

Sleeve prep:

Holding the two arches of the right foot, as above, have the recipient rotate the end of the foot to the inside, then wait (this is not a circle; you are turning the foot inward, in the direction the other foot. Practitioner, ease the tissues in the same direction as if rolling a ball slightly forward to be congruent with the bone of the foot. Wait. Recipient, rotate back to neutral. Wait. Practitioner, come to neutral. Wait. Repeat this procedure to the outside, then compare the two feet by moving them around gently. Go on to the mobilization work.

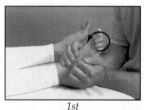

1st

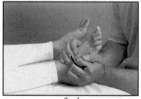

2nd

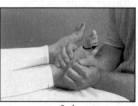

3rd

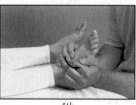

4th

Begin to alternate subtle pressure on first one arch then the other, upward toward the pelvis. Visualize the differentiation as it travels upward. The differentiation of the arches enhances the inner space, composed of membranes and nerves. These tissues send information upward and downward.

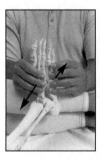 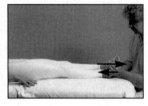 Gently grasp the base of the toes (where they meet the metatarsals) with one hand and the heel with the other.

Traction apart, gently taking up the slack in the membranes. This action engages the plantar membranes (the plantar apinerosis) and starts to engage the core of the foot tissues that run longitudinally directly through the arch, surrounding the talus (a central bone that is designed and positioned to receive the weight from the ground going upward and the tibia coming 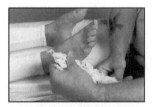 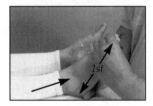 downward), and into the interosseous membrane. In essence, now you have a hold on the core membrane of the leg, including the talus.

Begin to traction downward, using the entire extended foot as a handle to reach up into the leg and beyond. You are fishing with the membranes of the lower leg for the contact with the pelvis. Using very fine line to get a bigger fish takes skill and sensitivity. You risk losing the connection.

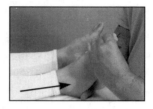

Once you've engaged the pelvis (use your felt sense; tracking through membranes is subtle yet very real. Put your mind in there and get your client to join you. It is about consciousness, use it!) slowly release, allowing the natural upward extension and span to take place. Play the fish, providing slack in the freshly connected membranes, permitting all the structures along the line of connection to disseminate and span or drift more freely within their comfort zone. Repeat the traction and release another time, then release slowly and return to neutral. Have recipient expose differences between the two feet; then do the other leg.

Now you have a good functional interaction between the information from the ground and the structures above. If you have done the other treatments the ball-and-sockets and outriggers of the foot and lower leg much integration is beginning to take place and the upper three cylinders are ready for further release. The following work can be done by you with or without the assistance of a partner. It is particularly helpful to have a self-integration section of each treatment to enhance the fact that the recipient did it, not the therapist. May I remind you that if the work is being offered within the principles of the Life Impressions process, the recipient is indeed doing all their own work with you as a guide.

Self Integration Phase

Main Cylinder Release Treatment

Have the recipient (or yourself, if you are practicing this on your own) on his back with knees up. Note which area receives the most or least pressure: the back of the head, the lowest part of the back (the sacrum), or the heels of the feet. Ask if the pressure is equal or more to one side of the body than another. (In short, fill in the self-image. If you know how you are, then you may have an opportunity to make change... a variation of an idea from Moshe.)

Note how the impressions change by pressing lightly on just the right heel. Track all the points we have mentioned. Release slowly. Do this several times, feeling how the movement travels up to the head. Does it come up evenly or more to one side? Extend legs and rest.

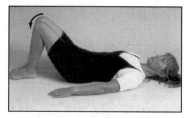 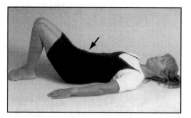

Bring the legs up to the standing position again feet flat on table as if they were standing and note impressions. Are things different? Scan carefully all the points of contact (there are many contact points, such as the shoulders, ribs, and so on). Begin to press gently with the right side of the sacrum, very gently, so that if someone were watching from above, they couldn't see any movement. Feel what happens to the impressions in the head and heels. Do they get heavier or lighter, is it different on one side than the other? Do this several times very slowly. Rest in neutral with the legs down. Scan and compare differences.

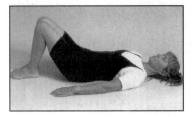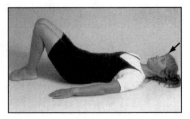

Resume beginning position. Now explore, very gently pressing the right side of the head into the floor or table. Note what happens in the spine. Are there some vertebra that move up toward the throat, and some that move in other directions? What happens in the sacrum? Is it the same on both sides when moving? Do this movement several times. Can you feel a response in the heels? Do all the movements on the left side, then rest, but remain in knee-bent position.

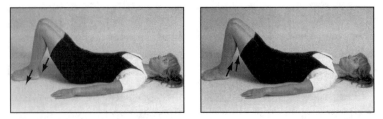

Press both heels gently downward and slightly away; rock gently, toward and away from the head (just slightly exaggerating the pressure on the floor, then releasing with a very slight lift on the feet will create the exaggeration).

Photos of heels, and rocking the whole body

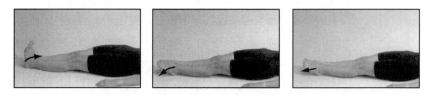

Notice how the movement travels up through the spine toward the cranium. Do this several times, resting in between. If you find an area that seems to be congested, see if you can find a way to send the movement to that area, using foot pressure and release. As the pressure increases on the area, consider that the awareness is increasing; don't try to make the area change physically. Awaken yourself to the area, that is enough. All this work is about awareness, not just mechanical action. As you slowly let the pressure off the heels, notice the movement of the entire spine downward toward the pelvis.

In the same position, shift your attention to the pelvis, slowly bringing the pubic bone up toward the chin. Notice how this movement travels through the spine and to the legs. Come back to neutral with the pelvis, then move the pubic bone down toward the feet, again following the movement. Continue to move the pelvis up and down, noting rib and head participation. Rest with knees down.

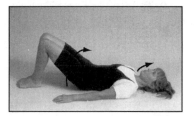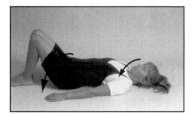

Return to the knees-up position and gently explore rocking the head in a "yes" motion. Note how much of the body is joining the movement. Rest, get up slowly and walk, noting differences.

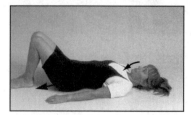 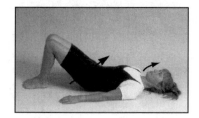

This "midline integration," or main cylinder treatment, is a fine completion to the outrigger treatment. It can also be a supplemental release for the body on its own.

KEYSTONE STRUCTURES TREATMENT

There are certain structures in the human body which are so closely related to other structures that, by their very position in the system, they have a great influence on how the organism as a whole will function. I call these keystone structures. The keystone is the central, topmost stone of an arch, or an essential part of a physical structure. I use keystone to refer to a structure which is central to many functional parts, that touches or relates intimately to all other parts in many actions.

For example, the sacrum is a keystone bone: it directly touches the spine above and the ileum on either side; it is directly connected to many lower viscera, literally surrounded by the nervous system and to some degree penetrating it. Through membranes, the sacrum is connected to the front and sides of the pelvis. In Ayurvedic medicine, the sacrum is considered the seat of the soul. That's quite a connection! The cerebral spinal fluid, which in Ayurveda is the carrier of the spiritual waters, or Kundalini, has a reservoir in the sacrum. Through its many direct and indirect connections, the sacrum, which rests at the center of the back of the pelvis, is an essential component both energetically, structurally, and functionally in the human organism.

The same is true of the occipital bone in the center of the back of the cranium, the sternum in the middle of the chest, the patella (knee cap) in the center of the leg, and the calcaneus at the center of the back of the foot. Without going into a detailed anatomical relationship of all the keystone structures, suffice it to say they all have, like the sacrum, a relationship to all structures around them. In my experience, if the keystone structures are subtly mobilized, they have a very positive influence on their associated structures. It's like pulling the rip cord on a parachute; if the parachute wasn't well-packed, the parachute won't blossom but will create a disorganized snarl. With well-done, non-invasive treatment of keystone structures, the whole system can blossom into full easy function.

The following procedure should be undertaken prior to the keystone treatment. By doing so, the more superficial outer layers of tissues, which might be patterned in a manner that could bind as the keystone structures emerge, can be resolved before the unraveling actions begin.

(1) Before the keystone treatment work, do the five vital air treatments in order to awaken and begin to reorganize the directional information inherent in the organism and its tissues, clearing the way for the keystone structures to emerge and continue the job of integration.

(2) Perform the outrigger treatments, including the sleeve work, to increase lateral support, safety, and begin to encourage differentiation of the layers of the system. Spanning the outriggers will begin the dehydration of the layers in the system, and thereby offer flexibility and an ability to sustain and respond to positive change.

(3) After the directional pathways are enhanced by the five vital air treatments and the structure is prepared, adding width and hydration between the layers, the keystone treatment using the principles of the Life Impression work and the Touch of Awakening can be very successful.

Remember that awareness is the healer; anytime you can awaken it, well-being can be increased.

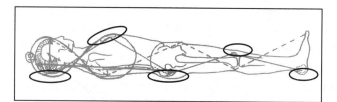

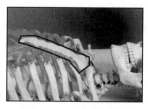

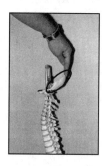

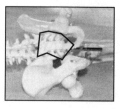

Note the figure-8 relationship of the keystone structures to their proximal body components and the soft tissue lacing that connects them. The keystone structures, from the top, are: the occipital bone, the sternum, the sacrum, the patella, and the calcaneus. Locate them on your own body and then on someone else's. Place your hand on a keystone bone and move it, noting how it responds and how adjunct structures interact. Because of inherent wisdom in these structures, this tracking of movement will be a big part of the treatment process. As the recipient receives tactile feedback regarding the actions relative to a given area, that area is highlighted in the awareness and can then be clarified and adjusted more easily for function.

The Keystone Treatment

The Occiput

Note: this treatment will follow the principles of the sleeve work you have already practiced.

Have the recipient lie on her back, legs extended. Observe, in "curious mode," the body with the keystone structures in mind. Notice any interesting patterns, rotations, side bending, depressions, etc., that you can see from this position around the areas of the keystone structures. You are not looking for what is wrong, just what is or is not functionally available.

Recall the relationship of the heels, pelvic, and cranial movements in the main cylinder treatment. Have the person slowly bring up her knees, watching how the system does or does not respond. Do this several times. Get feedback from the recipient about where she moves well and where there is restriction.

Place something under the knees to reduce the strain on the low back, and something small under the head (just enough to bring the head in line with the rest of the spine). Position yourself at the top of the body and place your hand under the head, fingers at the junction of the head and the spine, the base of the occipital bone. Your fingers should be precisely in the soft tissues at the base of the skull. Make sure your hand is in a comfortable place for the head to rest, as well as for you to be able to perceive clearly both position and any subtle changes. Your hand is not there to make change, but to offer feedback.

Have the person flex and extend the neck (drop the chin toward the chest then raise it, a "yes" motion). This movement must be very small; 1/4 inch at the most. Follow the movement of the tissues and bones under your fingers (you are clarifying and enhancing or increasing the neurological signal from the neck and its functional components). The more clearly one can feel what is or is not happening in the body, the more ability the recipient has to make positive changes. Follow the actions in both directions several times, emulating exactly the pattern they exhibit.

Recipient, raise the chin, then wait. Practitioner, bring the tissues up to match, wait. Recipient, return the chin to neutral. Wait a second, then come to neutral. Both parties wait. Once again, this delay differentiates the pattern of the tissues, allowing for new options to be included, and increases clarity of function. Do this several times, then stop in neutral.

Have the recipient tuck his chin (lower it toward the chest), and use the same delay technique, to match movement with the tissues. After the delay, follow with your hands as the occipital bone comes toward you, and stay there as the head returns to neutral. The practitioner also returns to neutral. This is all very gentle, so there should be no problem being able to slide the bone under your fingers. Become congruent with the recipients position at the neutral place. Do this several times.

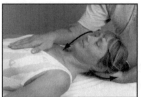

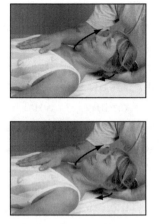

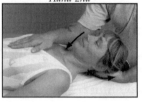

Hand Movement 1st
Hand 2nd

There are many more specific techniques for the area of the occipital but this will suffice for the pattern of treatment we are intending.

The Sternum

In this work we will consider the zyphoid, sternum, and manubrium as one, although in truth they can and do have potential to differentiate. There are further techniques for clarifying this specialized functional difference.

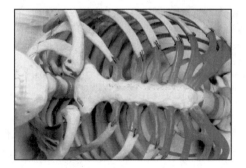

Position yourself at the person's head and spend a few moments observing the movement of the chest, particularly the area of the sternum. Place your hand on the sternum and follow its movements precisely as it moves with the breath. Be very specific. Follow any rotation, side bending, or whatever as clearly as you can; be a kinesthetic sounding board. Be careful not to get into leading. As you track the pattern, you want to observe and feed back to the person only what he or she is doing. What they do may change subtly as you increase the signal to their nervous system and you must change accordingly. Remember these original movements so you can compare after treating the area!

Explore the mobility of the sternum as if it were a boat on the water. Gently press its edges into the water, in this case the bodily waters of the tissues and joint fluids. Where does it sink most easily? Where is there some resistance to the pressure?

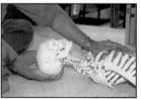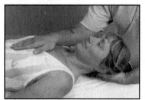

Basic Following Position

Repeat the easiest pattern of movement and hold gently for several breaths, then release on an inhalation. Explore the diagonals by squishing the manubrium and the zyphoid edges (we are treating them as part of the sternum) into the water element. Once again, note the areas that sink with ease. Repeat the pressure on the easy corners and hold for several breaths.

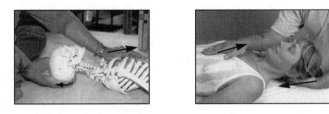

Ease the sternum downward toward the pelvis, then upward toward the head. Repeat the easiest pathway several times and then hold for a few breaths; release on the inhalation.

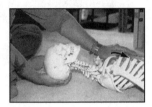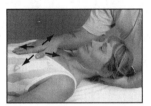

Re-test as you did at the beginning; note changes, have recipient note changes in breath, general thoracic cage awareness. Quite often the cylinders begin to ease apart with the breath. Ask if there is more clarity of movement between each rib and if the back of the cage can be felt.

Often positive changes, such as you may have cultivated at this point, will be tentative because they are new and the rest of the system is in an older pattern and basically uninformed as to the change. A clear sense of self, perceiving self-image accurately, will lead to functional options, or an ability to change in other ways. Integration is the key to enhancing the assimilation of the work. One of the best methods of integration is movement, particularly movement instigated in the areas of the current ease that has been developed.

Integration Occiput to the Sternum

Have the recipient rest on the back with knees up, feet standing, Place one hand under the head holding the occiput passively and the other hand on the sternum. Have the person repeat the main cylinder movement, rocking from the head, then from the pelvis with the head in the "yes" motion. As they do so, follow and slightly enhance the actions of those two structures in the movement. Pay attention to responsive actions in the chest and sternal area. Have the recipient rest in neutral; note the entire body for changes.

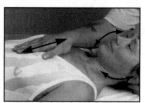

Include Pelvic Motion

The Sacrum

Work while person is on the back, placing your hand under the pelvis to monitor and treat the following.

Place one hand under the sacrum and the other on the sternum. Observe the movements of the sacrum as it

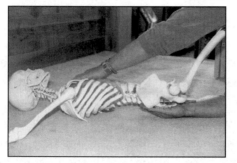

rides on the breath. If the system is reasonably well-organized, there will be movement through the spine and diaphragm that will express itself in the movement of the lumbar vertebra and the sacrum. Note movements that seem one-sided, such as a slide to one corner, or excessive downward movement with very little upward exertion. Relative to what you feel, ask what the recipient feels to see if you are congruent with what his body is expressing. (No judgment is needed here; curiosity is your best therapeutic tool in this type of exploration.) Don't be concerned if you are not congruent with your perceptions; this just indicates room for learning and change.

Continuing with the hand under the sacrum, ask the person to tuck his tail under very slightly, then lift it toward the ceiling. This must be a very gentle small movement. Follow the movement a few times, then exaggerate the dominant action. For example, if the bone moves up more easily, enhance that. You are not fixing anything; that is the recipients job.

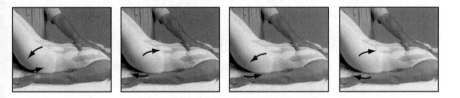

Have the recipient stop the movement and rest. Monitor at neutral, again noting any change. Go back to an active phase by having the person move the tail, monitoring with your hand. Once again choose the direction of ease and slightly enhance that pathway. Return to neutral.

Have the recipient turn onto the back, and repeat the integration movement, otherwise known as the Main Cylinder Integration. This time initiate from the pelvis to get the

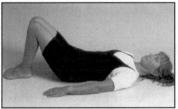

Rock from pelvis, then from the head

head and sternum involved. Then, rock whole body from heals.

The Patella and Calcaneus

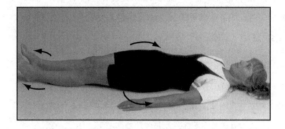

Recipient on the back with legs extended on the table. Have her bend one knee at a time and notice any variation from side to side. Ask for feedback. Does she note a difference? If so, is it what you see? How does the foot act in the movement? Is that the same side to side?

Focus on just one leg. Familiarize yourself with how the leg bends, then take that action over for the recipient. By taking over I mean support entirely and help her follow through with the movement. After two or three following passes through the action, have the recipient be completely passive and continue to do the movement for her as best you can. Make the movement very small. Note how far the knee rotates out or in, how much the ankle bends, and so on. Copy this action as perfectly as you can without the recipients active help in the movement. By taking over the pattern of action, the recipient can "listen more and effort less," with the result being that the nervous system gets clearer feedback as to what is happening.

How to take over the limb: slide one hand under the

knee, place the other in the joint of the ankle (top side). A second option: lay the other forearm across the bottom of the foot. From this support position, follow the movement, then take over while the recipient becomes passive. Lift under the knee, only about two or three inches. If you lift too far, the foot will begin to track behind and the joint actions between the knee and ankle will be disrupted. Follow the bend and the rotations of the femur, as well as the joint action of flexion and extension between the tibia and the talus (a saddle joint). The calcaneus gets a feeling of how it drops backward during this activity. Once again you are priming the pump, refreshing the memory of how the joints work together, without effort, which enhances the functional ability and the personal understanding and identification with the action.

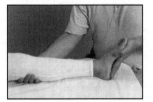 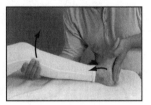

Take the limb through these actions many times, then rest in neutral. Have the recipient compare the actions of the two limbs. Do the other limb in the same manner.

Keystone Integration

Recipient on back with something under the knees like a rolled-up towel, just enough to raise the knees two to three inches. Have the person begin to rock the heels, sending the movement upward through the head. Keep the action going, switching the area that is generating the movement from the heels to the pelvis, pelvis to the head and then back down. This movement, coupled with your treatment, will offer a great sense of connectedness. The main cylinder movement that has been laced throughout the treatment can be used to refresh the functional memory.

Chapter Ten

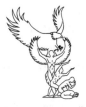

Elemental Treatments

Before we delve into more treatments using manual techniques, please remember there are many effective treatment pathways one can use for elemental imbalances, such as herbs, diet, and cleansing processes (see Resources). In general, any change in the organism or emotions will initiate a change in the elements, so whenever you are treating anything, you are treating elementally. With more specific "elemental" treatments such as the ones which follow, you must consider the attributes of the predominant elements or dosha towards which you are directing your treatment.

The treatments in the last few chapters may have seemed Western in their manner of description, but they also tend to the "elemental system" as well as the seven layers of tissues, the dhatus. Any change in the organism affects the entire being on all levels. We may think we are just moving a bone in the foot, but if we are doing it in an acceptable manner for the person receiving the contact, all levels will be receiving "notice of change." Think of a pebble dropped into the pool of your being: "effect" ripples will travel outward. As the ripples move outward in a pond, the sandy sediment at the bottom is slightly disturbed, as would be our earth elements; the microbes in the pond will ride the wave action, as will the particles in the blood (rasa) and lymph (rakta) in the human body. A tadpole may have to wiggle its tail to deal with the liquid movement; in the human form, somewhere along the line from the foot action, the fluid and mechanical transmission of movement may move your kidney. My point is that we have already been doing elemental treatments, although using Western terminology.

As we now look more into specific elemental treatments, remember that the mechanical actions will also be responding. This translation again is made possible through awareness and the inter-relationship of all the components of the system via the nervous system, the connecting membranes, the skeleton, and the fluids.

The following elemental treatments are designed for the notable element that may be outstanding, or out of relationship to the others. You might say these are treatments for the individual constitutional type, but remember each of us is made of all the elements; under certain conditions, we who are kapha types may find ourselves vata deranged, pitta or fire people may have an experience that enhances their emotions to the point were they are water deranged, and so on. Therefore, don't rule out the potential need for any of these treatments for all the constitutions.

Although I am giving some directives regarding specific treatment sessions, the purpose of this book is to give you enough information and tools so you may begin to read the "living book" and learn to build treatments around immediate needs.

Vata Excess

The symptoms of excess vata are: dryness of the skin and other body parts, coldness, rough skin, a very delicate nature, excessive nervous movements, constipation, pain in the pelvic bones, dry cracking joints, and fear and anxiety. Some of the qualities attributed to kapha and pitta will help to balance excess vata, such as: unctuousness (oiliness), warmth, softness, stability, heaviness and stillness of the nerves. Since an increase of vata produces an increase in fear, a feeling of safety is of primary importance. Slow small movements and, in some cases, just holding without movement can help quiet the nervous system. In preparation for the treatment, the environment should be warm, quiet, and comforting, establishing immediately a degree of sedation and safety.

According to Ayurveda, the torso is generally divided elementally: the lowest section of the abdomen near the pelvis is primarily vata, the mid-section is primarily pitta, and the chest is basically kapha. The main locations of vata in the body are the colon, lower back, ears, bones, and skin. All these locations need to be very mobile, thus the need for additional air and ether, the mobile elements. One factor to consider in the treatment of vata is that excess movement increases vata, therefore these areas are the most likely to become vata-deranged before the problem shows up in other areas.

Relative to other parts of the functional anatomy, the legs are more vata-genic (more energetic and mobile), therefore we begin the treatment at the feet. If you recall the nature of the air and ether elements that constitute vata, they tend to disperse in the system, leaving the individual somewhat ungrounded, lacking stability and strength. Working on the feet will help ground and increase security as well as help direct the needed vata energy into the legs. The level of the work is primarily on the bone layer (asthi dhatu) and the nerve tissues (majji dhatu). Bone is one of the locations of vata, therefore it must be tended in order to bring vata back into balance.

Remember that cold, dryness, and movement increase vata. Receiving bodywork can increase movement as the body opens it may become cold and the tissues may absorb all the moisture on the surface. In this treatment we treat sedatively as we progress through the steps. Drinking boiled milk with some fresh ground peppercorn and honey will sedate, warm and nourish the system after the treatment. You may find it helpful to include the directional movements of the five vital airs as you do the work. On occasion, it will be included in the treatment itself.

Use warm oil (sesame oil is good for vata because it is slightly heating) to sedate the nervous system, and to counter-act the dry and rough qualities of vata. You may want to have a saucepan full of water on a very low flame with a plastic squeeze bottle of oil in it. If you don't use oil during the treat-ment, then apply it afterwards. The first part of this treatment works with the feet to increase support, add grounding, and sedate the nervous system.

Treatment for Vata Excess

Place recipient on his back with something under his knees and covered with a blanket (to increase warmth and security). Grasp the right foot with both hands and hold. Wait, be patient, give him the sense that you will be with him for as long as necessary. The first contact should indicate the intention of the treatment which is support, giving a sense of having clear boundaries, warmth from your hands, and calm (do not touch with an agenda, vata is so tactually sensitive it will immedi-ately perceive your intent).

Apply warm oil to the feet.

Position your hands so that you are holding the big toe with the fingers of one hand and the "root" of the toe between the metatarsal and the last filangial joint. Move the toe slowly, use very small movements, just enough for him to notice, (remember movement increases vata and we are interested in sedation). The toes represent the most distal end of the nervous system. Gentle movement will offer clarity of function, bio-mechanical and elemental transition of fluids and membranes, joint mobilization, neurological feedback and sedation, and enhancement of the flow of apana, which will help with grounding and stability and thus with safety and support. Can you imagine all this from just mobilizing the toes?

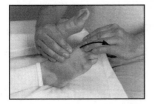 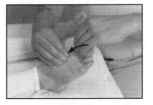

If you move slowly enough, the recipients breathing will change and he may even let out a relaxing sigh. This is a very simple technique, but if done correctly it can produce great relaxation and balance. Remember, it is not about technique; it is about awareness. You are cultivating awareness of gentle easy actions that are well-supported and contained. You are identifying a structural relationship that when clearly felt can be relied upon for support (this is particularly important when the vata is excessive). You are likely to have to contend with your own mind: "I should be doing more... this is slow... he must be bored... I am bored," and so on. In fact, a person suffering from an increase in vata will most likely be enjoying this simple experience.

Go through this same process with all the toes, mobilizing the third toe joint of each toe. When you complete the little toe, hold all the toes in a comforting manner.

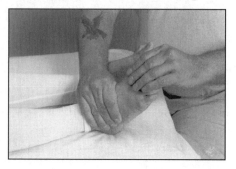

You are providing a better sense of a container. It is primarily kapha that makes up the containing membranes, so in a way you are enhancing the feeling of having some kapha and the support that it offers.

There are basically three transverse functional seams in the foot which are related to the torso structurally and energetically. If the "toe hinge" (the toe/metatarsal junction) is not being utilized, for whatever reason, there will be a dysfunctional area in the knee, the neck and upper thoracic area. Part of this relationship is set up structurally, and part is energetic, there is even an astrological relationship to all the body parts (aside from the fact that we are all one membrane and thus everything is related to everything else in the organism). When there is functional difficulty in the "hinge of the toes," which there often is with increased vata, the sensory nerves that connect that area of our body to the upper body do not recognize that the forward part of the foot is "there," providing support. The upper body area begins to contract and attempts to lever itself up, the nervous system is aggravated at having to work overtime, and vata increases. If this happens for some time, the cervical thoracic area becomes an island unto itself through its self-contained efforts, further isolating it from support and from the toe hinge. In essence, the two related areas cancel themselves out by over-functioning for their own ends, simply because they cannot sense one another. The same response happens between the tarso-metatarsal joints and the lumbar-thoracic area of the torso, and the transverse tarsal joints and their counterpart above in the lumbar-sacral area.

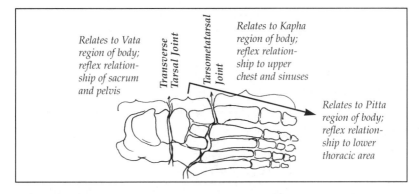

Relates to Vata region of body; reflex relationship of sacrum and pelvis

Transverse Tarsal Joint

Tarsometatarsal Joint

Relates to Kapha region of body; reflex relationship to upper chest and sinuses

Relates to Pitta region of body; reflex relationship to lower thoracic area

Much of our treatment for vata excess has to do with reconnecting all the body parts so that none are overworked, insecure or vulnerable (traits of increased vata). It's all about the relationship we have with ourselves being able to "feel" our self-image both physically and energetically. If we can access a body part, we can continually make the needed corrections; if not, we fall down and can't get up, or increase nervous energy to superficially sustain ourselves at great expense to our energy savings account. Now back to our story. Our hero has the recipient on the table and has just completed the infamous toe wiggling...

With the fingers of one hand, begin at the small toe side of the foot by holding the distal metatarsal head; with the other hand, make contact and stabilize at the tarso-metatarsal "seam." Move the bone (metatarsal) from the distal end (the toe end) very slowly, and just a tiny bit, in a flexion/extension movement. Then proceed through each metatarsal in the same manner.

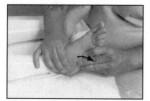 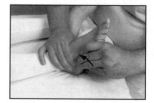

You are re-introducing the recipient to this area of his anatomy. Through the distal movement of the metatarsal, you are directing his attention and mobilizing the tarso-metatarsal "seam," which has a very strong relationship, both structurally and energetically, to the area where the lumbar and thoracic vertebra meet. This area also relates to the kidney and adrenal area of the body, and these organs can be positively affected by working on the foot. This area of the foot tends to be one of the most unused or misused structures of the foot. Frequently this is the case with the corresponding areas of the spine and ribs from the mid-thoracic to the upper-lumbar area. The two combined areas are very often lost or held back from full participation in the actions of the human system and this creates overwork in other areas, again increasing stress and vata. This treatment can begin to awaken these areas so they may be included in the awareness and function, increasing support and reducing vata.

Work gently. If the organism senses a challenge, an inner alarm goes off, safety is questioned, the nervous system calls for protection, which increases vata and compromises the treatment. Vata imbalance is responsible for 60% of all dis-ease. You need not have a vata constitution to need this treatment.

Remember, however, that the kapha person needs to become active after sedation of any kind.

You may want to add more warm oil to the foot now.

Anchor the space between the index finger and the thumb of the hand at the transverse tarsal joint or seam and mobilize the bones distal to it, beginning with the cuboid on the big toe side of the foot, then the navicular, then the three cuneiform bones.

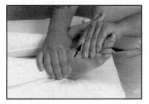 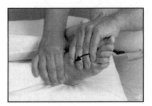

Increased mobility at the transverse tarsal seam, when offered subtly, can awaken and release the lumbar area of the back and stabilize the pelvis. The pelvis and low abdomen are a major location for vata, therefore this is a great place to sedate and balance. The use of the warm oil, the gentleness of the treatment and the location of the treatment all will help to reduce vata.

To complete the foot work we offer oleation therapy. Apply the warm oil to bottom of the foot, then wrap with a towel. This procedure nourishes the tissues, sedates vata, lubricates the joints and seams, and calms the nerves. Do the other foot, then wrap it.

We continue the treatment working now on the abdomen to sedate vata, settle the peristaltic actions, and stabilize the low back.

Continuing from the foot work, keep the feet covered and warm, and the knees bent to relax the abdominal muscles. Sit on the right side of the person with the

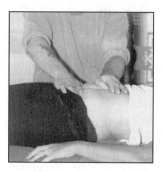

warm oil at your disposal. Place your hands on the right side of the abdomen, the right hand on the inside of the ileum near the pubis (find the hollow created by the pelvic bone). Place the left hand on the right side of the abdomen just below the rib cage.

Picture in your mind the envelope that contains the organs, how it fills out the bony container made of the pelvic bones, the rib cage, and the spine. Scoop out the masonry envelope from under the bones on the right side of the body.

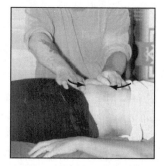

This is very gentle. You are offering the envelope and your hands as support to the organs on the right side, particularly the ascending colon (a major location of vata). As if you were cradling a baby, surround the ascending colon and other organs in that area of the pelvis, just slightly lifting it by using the heel of your hand and the thumb. Maintain this support for several breaths. This gives the person time to feel safe and the organs time to relax further. Then ease off back to where neutral will now be.

Here again it is very common for people to sigh with relief when this technique is done well. Your support reduces anxiety, increases stability, frees up the fluids that surround the organ itself and the organ cavity, and can sedate the nervous system. But your contact must be very gentle. Even though I do not always indicate it, you are encouraged to use the step-by-step Touch of Awakening procedure: make contact, listen, follow, then either exaggerate or follow the pattern of the treatment indicated, then return to neutral.

Another way of looking at the work is that through your contact you are giving the area of treatment a taste of its present position and condition. By enhancing this and adding support, you are providing the recipients nervous system with information which can lead to an increase in support and safety, mobilization of the tissues, and a gradual unraveling of the area.

Leave your left hand where it is and replace your right hand on the left side of the body just under the rib cage. Hold and wait for the nervous system to catch up and give approval. Draw your hand and the contained structures 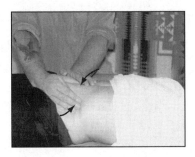 together very slightly (maybe 1/4 of an inch) and hold for several breaths, then release.

Ease both hands off the body and have the person breathe softly, noticing the change. Still seated on the right side, place your left hand just under the rib cage on the left, place the right hand just above the pelvic bones on the left, and gather the tissues off the lateral wall of

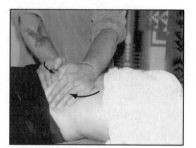

the body and out of the bony corners. Hold, then release slowly.

Cover the abdomen while you get the warm oil, then uncover and apply the oil to the entire abdomen, using a clockwise motion from the navel outward. Do not rub it in, just offer a coating of oil, then cover and keep warm while the oil soaks in. Note: if the recipients digestion is very poor, do not use oil as it may be difficult to assimilate into the system.

To complete this treatment, you may add a few drops of warm oil in the nostrils and in the ears; you may also treat the hands in the same manner that you did the feet, apply oil and cover to keep warm.

Following the treatment, the vata person should remain quiet, drink warming liquids like ginger tea, take a hot bath followed by application of warm oil, wrap up in a fluffy robe, breathe slowly several times through the right nostril while closing off the left, then meditate deeply.

PITTA EXCESS

Possible symptoms of excess pitta include: heat, hyper-toned tissues, redness of the skin, headaches, pressure in the head, anger, impatience, tightness in the chest, redness in the eyes, impatience, and anger. With these symptoms in mind, consider how to balance the system, what elements to add, how to touch, and so on.

The main locations of pitta in the body are under the skin (to maintain body temperature), in the liver, the small intestine, the gray matter of the brain, and the eyes. Heat tends to move upward, in the outer as well as the inner environment. With an increase in pitta, there will certainly be heat rising. It can be very dangerous for too much heat to accumulate in the upper cavities of the body, especially the head, so the first thing we want to do is reduce heat in the head.

For the pitta person (especially when the pitta is in excess), it is very important to work in a manner that causes little or no friction, as friction will increase the systemic heat under the skin. For this treatment we will introduce the "pocketing" stroke a manual technique that gets under the surface layer (where pitta is located). By getting just under the pitta layer, one may access the interstitial fluids and adipose tissues (yes, even pitta has some) and cool the skin by hydrating it. The treatment environment should be a cool room, with the shades drawn. A person with increased pitta will have a sensitivity to light. Soothing music can be helpful. Cooling colors, such as blue or purple, can be helpful.

Treatment for Excess Pitta

Begin the treatment with the person on her back, and place a cool cloth on the forehead (you might soak it in some cooling Aloe Vera juice or mint tea). A cool cloth behind the neck may also be helpful. Place slices of cucumber on the eyelids.

With the recipient on her back with knees bent, feet standing, begin to focus on the pitta zone from about the navel to the diaphragm. Grasp the abdominal muscles with both hands on either side of the navel, scoop and lift off the underlying tissues. Have the person breathe gently into the area. Too strong a breath will push you out. With some people, the abdominal area can be very tight; do not force yourself under the muscles, just gather what you can. You may have to pocket the tissues holding with one hand while the other slides under the abdominals. (See second illustration.) You are "ventilating" the fire region –don't work to change the structure, use consciousness.

As the rectus abdominus muscle is lifted off the organs (particularly the small intestine where pitta is stored), the fluids about the viscera rush into the space created and can act as a coolant, sedating pitta. Also, the excess pitta contained in the small intestine can be moved out through the natural enhancement of the visceral activity, set in motion by the release of compression offered by this stroke. Rest, then have the person breathe, noting the difference. Do the stroke again. If this is done well, there will be a noticeable sense of ease upon breathing into the area after the stroke is released.

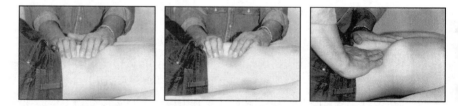

On the right side is the liver (another repository of liquid fire in the body) and behind that is the gallbladder (a storage facility for the bile, considered fire in the Ayurvedic system). The whole diaphragm area is often tight when there is an excess of pitta. Place your hands on either side of the rib cage near the bottom where the diaphragm attaches to the back side of the lower rib cage. Note the available squish by pressing slightly inward just enough to take up the slack in the ribs relative to the underlying tissues, compress only 1/8th inch. Rotate your hands about an inch, hold, and have the person breathe into your hands.

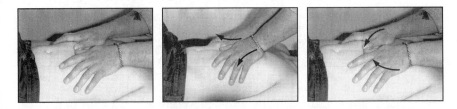

Slowly rotate the other way. Have recipient again breathe into your hands. Slowly release your hold. Remove your hands and let her explore the change. This can be very powerful for the pitta, indicating just how much is held in the area and giving support so that the holding may be released. Changes can occur in the strain pattern in the ribs, and the underlying organs of the liver and gallbladder may be mobilized.

Place the hands on the rib cage in the same place, but this time squish downward toward the pelvis, again only about 1/8 to 1/4 inch. The contact you offer must be very slight. You will get much more change with a gentle touch. In essence, pitta under the diaphragm is a powder keg. Don't set off the charge. You might want to follow this treatment

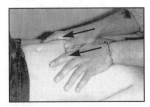

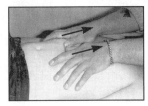

with enhancement of the prana and apana vital airs.

Remove the cucumbers from the eyes. Put two cotton balls in some cold milk and place in the refrigerator to be used after the following treatment application.

Place your fingers around the eyeball, gently, so that the orb is entirely surrounded. Begin to slightly pivot the orb upward. These actions are so slight that they are almost just an intention. Pivot back to center, stop a moment, pivot downward, back to center. Wait, then to the left, back and rest, to the right, back and rest. Do the diagonal corners in the same manner, resting in the middle.

Ease your hands off the eyes, then place the cotton balls on the eyelids. The support you have offered the eyes, and the assisted mobility, can release tension and accumulated heat; the milk-soaked cotton balls will draw out heat and soothe the eyes. (The recipient may gasp as the cold penetrates into the eyes.)

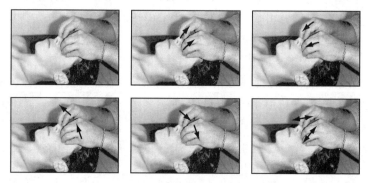

After treatment, suggest that the recipient take a cool shower, breathe a few times slowly and deeply through the left nostril while closing off the right (particularly when stress arises), drink some cool mint tea, and meditate.

Kapha Excess

Kapha accumulates in the sinuses, the lungs, the stomach, and the more massive tissues of the body. Symptoms which indicate the need for this treatment are: congestion, particularly in lungs and sinus, sluggishness; swelling and edema; dull aching pain; lethargy and depression; heaviness; and weight gain. These are all signs of a kapha constitution, but the same symptoms may be experienced by another constitutional type if they have developed a water imbalance. For example, if a vata person overeats and can't digest the food, the undigested food becomes kapha excess and possibly toxic, so a vata person can benefit from a kapha-reducing treatment under certain conditions. The design of this specific treatment is to reduce kapha, but as with all treatments, the session will not impose demands on the organism, only aid in restoring balance. Although organized to help in a particular manner, the work is always subservient to the wisdom of the organism. If the problem is acute, you may want to consult an appropriate medical expert.

Since kapha is cold by nature, the treatment environment should be warm but not stuffy, as this might cause drowsiness and more lethargy. If you play music, it should be somewhat lively to begin to move the stagnant energy from the inside out. If you use incense or essential oils, the fragrance should be something spicy and invigorating. With kapha, one should usually avoid using oils and instead use water or water-based cream if some lubrication is needed. If you do use oil, use calamus oil or sprinkle calamus powder on the body before applying oil.

Because kapha gathers in the fleshy parts of the body, we treat the large muscle groups, and access the membrane pumps. Because of the nature of the condition, we employ more tamasic and rajasic types of manual contact. Tamasic breaks up congestion and awakens, rajasic moves the fluids and unravels the tissue patterns. Basic Swedish massage is quite good for the excessive water condition.

Treatment for Reducing Kapha

Lower Limbs

Have the client lie on his back, knees supported with a pillow. Begin at the lower leg. Grasp the calf muscles firmly in both hands (you will have to be a little above the ankle so you are on the belly of the muscle), encapsulate the muscles, giving a sense of support, and wait for the structure to fall further into your palms. Once the muscles have oozed into your hand (kapha-laden tissues can definitely ooze), take the whole bundle upward to the extent that the membranes can yield or, you might say, take up the slack and hold there. This action differentiates the layers and opens the membrane space between the gastrocnemius muscle and the deeper layers for better fluid transfer.

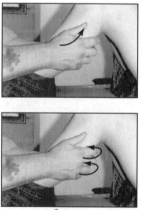

Squeeze

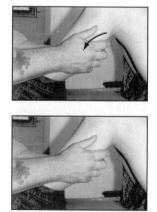

Reverse

Ask the recipient to move his ankle while you maintain your hold in the same position. This enhances the mechanical pumping action that moves the fluid. Stop the movement, and rhythmically squeeze the tissues in your hand the "sponge-wringing" rajasic technique. Follow with client-assisted pumping action again. Have recipient compare the two legs to enhance the neurological learning, then do the other lower leg in the same manner.

Between each manual technique, have the client breathe vigorously several times through the right nostril, which increases the heat in the system and begins to melt down the kapha so it is more easily eliminated or transmuted into vitality.

Recipient in the same position, slip your hands under the 'belly' of the thigh (the area of the most bulk, the hamstrings) and go through the process of supporting the tissues until they yield into your hand. You must wait for this, otherwise you are just doing mechanical manipulation. This is a process of communication. Interactive person-to-person work can offer learning as part of the transition; it is the learning that maintains and can reproduce the change.

After the hamstrings have been gathered, slide them as a group upward toward the pelvis. The upward movement counteracts the downward settling of the heavy elements. Do not move on the skin; carry the muscle group to a new place to offer awareness and functional differentiation. Hold in the up-side pattern, asking the recipient for gentle contraction and extension, such as a soft attempt to bend and straighten the knee.

Address the client's attention and place your own attention deep in the area between the bone and the layers of tissue under the hamstrings. Stop the movements, then alternately do the rajasic squeeze and relaxation. Feel you are helping him empty the excess water from the tissues, squeezing out a sponge. Ease off your support of the thigh and have him explore the difference leg to leg. Do other leg. Suggest that he walk after the treatment and encourage him to include more walking in his daily life. The legs will feel like walking after this treatment, and walking is the best exercise for moving all systems, particularly the fluid systems. Do the same procedure on the quadriceps on both legs. This same treatment can be applied to the arms.

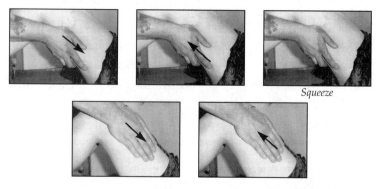

Squeeze

Another place that kapha accumulates is in the area of the stomach. Although there are very specific visceral manipulations that can be applied to each and every organ, we offer here a general treatment of the mesentery envelope. Treatment of this area is designed to mobilize the general digestive potential by addressing the container (the mesentery envelope itself).

The organs, like all other structures in the body, are contained and can become habitual in patterns of function which freeze the container in place. Also, like all tissues and functional systems in the human body, there is a balance of the elements that must be established. It's like adding too much water in a cake mix, which dilutes the flavor, cancels out the baking action, and slows the cooking process. As we work in the area of the viscera, consider that there is an interaction between all the organs. If they are flooded with too much liquid, or compressed in a smaller area due to fluid pressures about them, dysfunction is bound to occur. On the other hand, like all organic systems, if there is enough room to function and awareness is present, self-corrections and healing will take place. This is the purpose of the treatment in this area. Although disbursement of excess fluids may be needed, our goal is to awaken and enable the area to do what it knows how to do naturally.

Stomach

Place recipient on his back, legs supported. This position reduces the inferior pull on the pelvis and abdominal musculature, permitting the area to be more relaxed and receptive.

Sit at the side of the person near the midsection. Reach across the midline and find the lateral edge of the abdominal muscles (rectus abdominis). With all the fingers of both hands, press into the space between the rectus and the oblique, and slightly pull toward the midline. While holding the pull, have the client breathe into the area, infusing the area with more awareness and creating some functional change. The visceral envelope which lies under the abdominal muscles is freed from any excessive engagement to the surface structures.

This helps to clarify the functional seam between the two structures and define the functional position of the rectus muscle; if the rectus muscle is more clearly in the midline of the body, it works more efficiently to support the midline, taking any burden off the underlying tissues (when they don't have to protect against the outside environment, they can tend to the local business at hand, such as pumping fluid, etc.) As any structure becomes clearer in its position and function, others in the vicinity become clearer and more functional.

Work up and down the lateral edge to cover as much of the rectus as you can, having the client breathe into the area each time. After doing one side, have the recipient breathe into the abdomen several times, noting the difference from side to side. There is often a sense of lightness, which in itself begins to balance the heavy qualities of kapha. Do the other side in the same manner.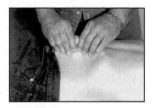

Stand at the head of the table and reach down over the abdomen, making contact just above the pubic bone with both hands parallel. Draw upward toward the head (get down to the level of the muscle if you can), take up the slack and hold. Ask the client to breathe into the lower abdomen several times, then release. Move your hands up to the next segment in the rectus abdominus, about an inch or two. Grasp there and pull upward, taking up the slack. Hold and have the client breathe several times again. Rest, then move up to the next muscle segment (you may need to approximate with some individuals). Continue in this manner until you reach the rib cage, then do one of the ribs (this is the superior attachment of the rectus abdominus).

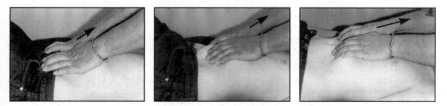

The support you offer with your hold and lift helps to differentiate the visceral bag from the bony container; the layer differentiation can enhance the functional activities of the organs and the tone of the tissues contained in the abdominal region. Because you are working in the area of the abdomen, you are also stimulating vata and pitta, both of which will be helpful to our kapha friend. The mesentery envelope is designed to contain and protect the organs; when it gets overly connected to the ribs or pelvis, its ability to care for the organs is impaired. Any time a structure begins to engage with more than one structure, its functional ability may be compromised. In fact, the organs themselves may be drawn off their axes of functional ease. For example, the gall bladder duct, a very small but important structure, can be disrupted by the rib cage imposing on it from above if there is not adequate gliding surface between the duct, the liver, the mesentery envelope, and the ribs. This may sound complex, but it is important to understand that your touch indeed has a specific useful action in the mechanical relationships in the body.

The chest is one of the main locations for kapha in the body. The muscles of the chest are large (in general, mass is composed of water and earth). The lungs, being water, are also kapha. Both can accumulate water very easily. The following treatment of the chest is designed to free congestion in both the muscles of the chest and enhance fluid exchange in the lungs and pericardium. The sternal work of the keystone treatment can also be used to access the mobility in the chest (the key to unlocking the chest mechanically). Increased mobility will counteract the static quality of kapha. Also, increased mobility often increases the ability of the tissues to break down congestion in the interstitial fluids. Herbs and other types of cleansing procedures may be necessary. Generally this treatment is safe and non-invasive for most people, but if you have any questions or the recipient has a history of major congestion in the area, better check with an appropriate medical practitioner first.

Chest

Have the recipient on his back with the legs elevated. Position yourself at the head of the person and place your hands on the upper chest, just below the clavicles and next to the sternum. You are on top of the pectoral muscles, which attach along the clavicle and at the lateral sternal edge. With this hand position, you can stabilize the tissues while the bones are moved on the breath, thus creating space for better function and fluid exchange.

Take up the slack in the tissues between the surface and the ribs underneath. Very slightly twist your hands away from the middle, hold there and ask the client to breathe several times, then release. Repeat with the twist toward the middle. There are many structural dynamics that can be enhanced from this place, but for now we are only interested in offering increased awareness and increasing fluid exchange.

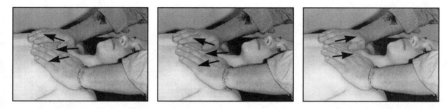

Working on the diaphragm and chest will separate the clinging tissues about the chest and under the diaphragm, move the fluids, increase respiratory response, and increase energy in the system. This in turn will counteract the attributes of congestion, staticity, heaviness, and coldness.

Follow the treatment by suggesting the kapha person should regularly take a vigorous walk while breathing deeply the entire time. Hot ginger tea will continue to break up congestion in the system. He should breathe through the right nostril while closing off the left vigorously, then meditate deeply. Take another walk, then rest.

This completes the treatment section of the book. Please realize what a task it is to convey something of a physical functional nature in words. Imagine, for example, writing down how to tie your shoe. For more ease of practice, please review as often as necessary, or make an audio tape of the instructions. You can also request both audio and video tapes from the Life Impressions Institute as aids for your work.

Once you feel comfortable with the treatments and the Touch of Awakening, trust in the principles of the work, understand the constitutional make-up of the person, and dispense with the aids. Listen in on the body telephone with your hands and heart!

Afterword

As a species, with the exception of a few saints, sages and an occasional genius, scientists tell us we use a very small proportion of our brains, about 15% of capacity. What potential we have for growth! The trick is knowing how to access this vast unused portion of our brain. Moshe Feldenkrais says if we can be aware of our non-habitual actions, this begins to open new aspects of our brain.

Developing new and different ways of functioning, acting, responding, and believing that are entered in an entirely new section of the brain would be like moving to a new country where no one knew us. In this new environment, in a new section of the brain, we could develop a new self-image. We could reframe our existence. If we added some deep contemplation and meditation on who we are, we could constantly be new and spontaneous and yet retain all the useful information we needed from our experiences.

If we update our old life impressions, utilize the Touch of Awakening, choose to really look at who we are from new perspectives, we can begin to use ourselves in different ways, think differently, begin to "see" ourselves as something or someone new and fresh all the time on all levels of our existence physical, emotional, mental, and spiritual. I hope that the information and practices in this book are of some value in making this come true.

When I was doing intense manual labor in a steel mill, I once had a day dream: if I could just remain relaxed in a comfortable place inside myself, appropriate work would come to me. As an aspiring "yogi," I visualized myself sitting and meditating in a holy place, surrounded by flowers and pictures of saints. In my daydream, people would come by and ask for assistance: "Can you fix my window?" "Can you move this tree root for me?" "Can we talk about meditation?" "Would you rub my back?" I would do the things they asked, they would give me money, and we would both be very satisfied.

Here I am many years later and what do I do? I clean my treatment room, pray in it, put flowers around and maintain a pleasant environment both within myself and in the room. People come asking for assistance; I treat them and they give me money. What a dream come true! This dream is even better, in that I find ways for the person to do their own work, giving them more satisfaction, and we both continue to work on ourselves.

My point is that we can all do this no matter what we do in life. We can keep our inner and outer environments in good condition, free from negativity, 'sacred' in a manner of speaking, by updating our life impressions. Even in a big corporate office, our own work station can be environmentally healthy, both inside and out. I could have made the job in the steel mill more enriching through my inner work. I hope you have all received some inspiration and practical experience from the contents of this book to help make your environments a better place to work, live, and prosper.

I would like to finish as I began, by asking Ganesha to remove all obstacles from our path toward well-being and self-awakening. May the saints and sages of all the religions be with us as we pass through our journey in this drama of life, and may all your life impressions be flexible.

Bibliography

Barral & Mercier, *Visceral Manipulation*, Eastland Press., Chicago, IL, 1983.

Feldenkrais, Moshe, *Body Awareness as Healing Therapy* (The case of Nora), Somatic Resources, Frog Ltd., Berkeley, CA.

Feldenkrais, Moshe, *Awareness Through Movement*

Frawley, David, *Ayurvedic Healing*, Passage Press, Salt Lake City, UT, 1989.

Frawley, David, and Lad,Vasant, *The Yoga Of Herbs*, Lotus Press, Twin Lakes, WI, 1986.

Joshi, Sunil, *Ayurveda and Panchakarma*, Lotus Press, Twin Lakes, WI, 1997.

Keleman Stanley, *Emotional Anatomy*, Center Press, Berkeley, CA.

Kurtz, Ron, *Hakomi Therapy*, Life Rhythm, publishing, Mendocino, CA, 1990.

Lad, Vasant, *Ayurveda, The Science of Self Healing*, Lotus Press, Twin Lakes, WI, 1984.

Morningstar, Amadea, *The Ayurvedic Cookbook*, Lotus Press, Twin Lakes, WI, 1990.

Painter, Jack, *Deep Bodywork and Personal Development*, self-published through the Center for Release and Integration, 450 Hillside Ave., Mill Valley, CA, 1984.

Painter, Jack, *Technical Manual of Deep Holistic Bodywork* (see above)

Rolf, Ida P, *Rolfing: The Integration of Human Structure,*
Dennis-Landman Publishers, Santa Monica, CA.

Svoboda Robert, *Prakruti: Your Ayurvedic Constitution,*
Geocom Ltd. Publishing, Albuquerque, NM, 1988.

Tiwari, Maya, *Ayurveda, Secrets of Healing,* Lotus Press,
Twin Lakes, WI, 1995.

Upledger and Vredevoogd, *Craniosacral Therapy,*
Eastland Press, Seattle, WA, 1983.

Resources

Life Impressions Institute
Donald VanHowten, Director
613 Kathryn Street
Santa Fe, New Mexico 87501
(505) 988-2627

Classes and Training Seminars

At the Institute, Donald VanHowten and staff offer short
and long-term classes in the Life Impressions bodywork
process. These classes are given at our location in Santa Fe, as
well as in other areas. Those who complete all classes can
become certified by the Institute. For information and complete details, send for our free brochure.

Practitioner Listings

A certified practitioner listing, from around the world, can
be obtained by contacting the Intitute.

Audio and Video Tapes Available

Recordings of the treatments and exercises in the book are
available upon request from the Institute. Please ask for a listing of tapes and price list.

Bodywork Training

The Life Impressions Institute
613 Kathryn Street
Santa Fe, NM 87501

The Center For Release and Integration
450 Hillside Drive
Mill Valley, CA 94941

Dr. Jay Scherer's Academy of Natural Healing
1443 St. Francis Drive
Santa Fe, NM 87505.

The Rolf Institute
205 Canyon Blvd.
Boulder, CO 80302

The Upledger Institute
11211 Property Farms Rd.
Palm Beach Gardens, FL 33410

The Feldenkrais Guild
524 Ellsworth St. SW, PO Box 489
Albany, OR 97321-0143

Ayurveda Centers and Programs

American Institute of Vedic Studies
P.O. Box 8357
Santa Fe, NM 87504-8357
(505) 983-9385
(505) 982-5807 (Fax)

The Ayurvedic Institute
11311 Menual N.E.
Albuquerque, NM 87112
(505) 291-9698
(505) 294-7572 (Fax)

Rocky Mountain Ayurvedic Health Retreat
P.O. Box 5192
Pagosa Springs, CO 81147
(800) 247-9654
(970) 264-9224

Vinayak Ayurveda Center
2509 Virginia, NE
Albuquerque, NM 87110
(505) 296-6522
(505) 298-2932 (Fax)

Ayurvedic Herbal Suppliers

Bazaar of India Imports, Inc
1810 University Avenue
Berkeley, CA 94703
(800) 261-7662

Internatural
33719 116th Street-AL
Twin Lakes, WI 53181,
(800) 643-4221
(Retail mail order supplier of Ayurvedic books and
herbal products.)

Kanak
P.O. Box 13653
Albuquerque, NM 87192-3643
(505) 275-2469

Lotus Brands, Inc.
P.O. Box 325-AL
Twin Lakes,WI 53181
(414) 889-8561
(414) 889-8591 (Fax)

Lotus Light
P.O. Box 1008-AL
Silver Lake, WI 53170
414-889-8501 or 800-548-3824
(414) 889-8591 (Fax)

General Healing Books and Inspirational Material

Metaphysical Meditations, Paramahansa Yogananda, Self Realization Fellowship, 3880 San Rafael Ave., Los Angeles, CA 90065

Scientific Healing Affirmations, Paramahansa Yogananda, Self Realization Fellowship

(All the many books by this great saint impart the power to heal yourself. Please contact the SRF organization.)

Index